全国中医药行业高等教育"十四五"规划教材

全国高等中医药院校规划教材（第十一版）

护理专业英语

（新世纪第四版）

（供护理学专业用）

主 编 刘红霞 刘 娅

中国中医药出版社

·北 京·

图书在版编目（CIP）数据

护理专业英语 / 刘红霞，刘娅主编 . —4 版 . —北
京：中国中医药出版社，2021.6（2024.9重印）
全国中医药行业高等教育"十四五"规划教材
ISBN 978-7-5132-6803-5

Ⅰ . ①护…　Ⅱ . ①刘… ②刘…　Ⅲ . ①护理学—英语—
中医学院—教材　Ⅳ . ① R47

中国版本图书馆 CIP 数据核字（2021）第 052128 号

融合出版数字化资源服务说明

全国中医药行业高等教育"十四五"规划教材为融合教材，各教材相关数字化资源（电子教材、PPT 课件、
视频、复习思考题等）在全国中医药行业教育云平台"医开讲"发布。

资源访问说明

扫描右方二维码下载"医开讲 APP"或到"医开讲网站"（网址：www.e-lesson.cn）注
册登录，输入封底"序列号"进行账号绑定后即可访问相关数字化资源（注意：序列号
只可绑定一个账号，为避免不必要的损失，请您刮开序列号立即进行账号绑定激活）。

资源下载说明

本书有配套 PPT 课件，供教师下载使用，请到"医开讲网站"（网址：www.e-lesson.cn）认证教师身份后，
搜索书名进入具体图书页面实现下载。

中国中医药出版社出版

北京经济技术开发区科创十三街 31 号院二区 8 号楼
邮政编码　100176
传真　010-64405721
河北省武强县画业有限责任公司印刷
各地新华书店经销

开本 889 × 1194　1/16　印张 13.75　字数 537 千字
2021 年 6 月第 4 版　2024 年 9 月第 5 次印刷
书号　ISBN 978-7-5132-6803-5

定价　54.00 元
网址　www.cptcm.com

服 务 热 线　010-64405510　　微信服务号　zgzyycbs
购 书 热 线　010-89535836　　微商城网址　https://kdt.im/LIdUGr
维 权 打 假　010-64405753　　天猫旗舰店网址　https://zgzyycbs.tmall.com

如有印装质量问题请与本社出版部联系（010-64405510）

全国中医药行业高等教育"十四五"规划教材
全国高等中医药院校规划教材（第十一版）

《护理专业英语》
编 委 会

全国中医药行业高等教育"十四五"规划教材
全国高等中医药院校规划教材（第十一版）

专家指导委员会

名誉主任委员

余艳红（国家卫生健康委员会党组成员，国家中医药管理局党组书记、局长）

王永炎（中国中医科学院名誉院长、中国工程院院士）

陈可冀（中国中医科学院研究员、中国科学院院士、国医大师）

主任委员

张伯礼（天津中医药大学教授、中国工程院院士、国医大师）

秦怀金（国家中医药管理局副局长、党组成员）

副主任委员

王　琦（北京中医药大学教授、中国工程院院士、国医大师）

黄璐琦（中国中医科学院院长、中国工程院院士）

严世芸（上海中医药大学教授、国医大师）

高　斌（教育部高等教育司副司长）

陆建伟（国家中医药管理局人事教育司司长）

委　员（以姓氏笔画为序）

丁中涛（云南中医药大学校长）

王　伟（广州中医药大学校长）

王东生（中南大学中西医结合研究所所长）

王维民（北京大学医学部副主任、教育部临床医学专业认证工作委员会主任委员）

王耀献（河南中医药大学校长）

牛　阳（宁夏医科大学党委副书记）

方祝元（江苏省中医院党委书记）

石学敏（天津中医药大学教授、中国工程院院士）

田金洲（北京中医药大学教授、中国工程院院士）

仝小林（中国中医科学院研究员、中国科学院院士）

宁　光（上海交通大学医学院附属瑞金医院院长、中国工程院院士）

匡海学（黑龙江中医药大学教授、教育部高等学校中药学类专业教学指导委员会主任委员）

吕志平（南方医科大学教授、全国名中医）

吕晓东（辽宁中医药大学党委书记）

朱卫丰（江西中医药大学校长）

朱兆云（云南中医药大学教授、中国工程院院士）

刘　良（广州中医药大学教授、中国工程院院士）

刘松林（湖北中医药大学校长）

刘叔文（南方医科大学副校长）

刘清泉（首都医科大学附属北京中医医院院长）

李可建（山东中医药大学校长）

李灿东（福建中医药大学校长）

杨　柱（贵州中医药大学党委书记）

杨晓航（陕西中医药大学校长）

肖　伟（南京中医药大学教授、中国工程院院士）

吴以岭（河北中医药大学名誉校长、中国工程院院士）

余曙光（成都中医药大学校长）

谷晓红（北京中医药大学教授、教育部高等学校中医学类专业教学指导委员会主任委员）

冷向阳（长春中医药大学校长）

张忠德（广东省中医院院长）

陆付耳（华中科技大学同济医学院教授）

阿吉艾克拜尔·艾萨（新疆医科大学校长）

陈　忠（浙江中医药大学校长）

陈凯先（中国科学院上海药物研究所研究员、中国科学院院士）

陈香美（解放军总医院教授、中国工程院院士）

易刚强（湖南中医药大学校长）

季　光（上海中医药大学校长）

周建军（重庆中医药学院院长）

赵继荣（甘肃中医药大学校长）

郝慧琴（山西中医药大学党委书记）

胡　刚（江苏省政协副主席、南京中医药大学教授）

侯卫伟（中国中医药出版社有限公司董事长）

姚　春（广西中医药大学校长）

徐安龙（北京中医药大学校长、教育部高等学校中西医结合类专业教学指导委员会主任委员）

高秀梅（天津中医药大学校长）

高维娟（河北中医药大学校长）

郭宏伟（黑龙江中医药大学校长）

唐志书（中国中医科学院副院长、研究生院院长）

彭代银（安徽中医药大学校长）

董竞成（复旦大学中西医结合研究院院长）

韩晶岩（北京大学医学部基础医学院中西医结合教研室主任）

程海波（南京中医药大学校长）

鲁海文（内蒙古医科大学副校长）

翟理祥（广东药科大学校长）

秘书长（兼）

陆建伟（国家中医药管理局人事教育司司长）

侯卫伟（中国中医药出版社有限公司董事长）

办公室主任

周景玉（国家中医药管理局人事教育司副司长）

李秀明（中国中医药出版社有限公司总编辑）

办公室成员

陈令轩（国家中医药管理局人事教育司综合协调处处长）

李占永（中国中医药出版社有限公司副总编辑）

张峘宇（中国中医药出版社有限公司副总经理）

芮立新（中国中医药出版社有限公司副总编辑）

沈承玲（中国中医药出版社有限公司教材中心主任）

编审专家组

全国中医药行业高等教育"十四五"规划教材
全国高等中医药院校规划教材（第十一版）

组　长

余艳红（国家卫生健康委员会党组成员，国家中医药管理局党组书记、局长）

副组长

张伯礼（天津中医药大学教授、中国工程院院士、国医大师）

秦怀金（国家中医药管理局副局长、党组成员）

组　员

陆建伟（国家中医药管理局人事教育司司长）

严世芸（上海中医药大学教授、国医大师）

吴勉华（南京中医药大学教授）

匡海学（黑龙江中医药大学教授）

刘红宁（江西中医药大学教授）

翟双庆（北京中医药大学教授）

胡鸿毅（上海中医药大学教授）

余曙光（成都中医药大学教授）

周桂桐（天津中医药大学教授）

石　岩（辽宁中医药大学教授）

黄必胜（湖北中医药大学教授）

前 言

为全面贯彻《中共中央 国务院关于促进中医药传承创新发展的意见》和全国中医药大会精神，落实《国务院办公厅关于加快医学教育创新发展的指导意见》《教育部 国家卫生健康委 国家中医药管理局关于深化医教协同进一步推动中医药教育改革与高质量发展的实施意见》，紧密对接新医科建设对中医药教育改革的新要求和中医药传承创新发展对人才培养的新需求，国家中医药管理局教材办公室（以下简称"教材办"）、中国中医药出版社在国家中医药管理局领导下，在教育部高等学校中医学类、中药学类、中西医结合类专业教学指导委员会及全国中医药行业高等教育规划教材专家指导委员会指导下，对全国中医药行业高等教育"十三五"规划教材进行综合评价，研究制定《全国中医药行业高等教育"十四五"规划教材建设方案》，并全面组织实施。鉴于全国中医药行业主管部门主持编写的全国高等中医药院校规划教材目前已出版十版，为体现其系统性和传承性，本套教材称为第十一版。

本套教材建设，坚持问题导向、目标导向、需求导向，结合"十三五"规划教材综合评价中发现的问题和收集的意见建议，对教材建设知识体系、结构安排等进行系统整体优化，进一步加强顶层设计和组织管理，坚持立德树人根本任务，力求构建适应中医药教育教学改革需求的教材体系，更好地服务院校人才培养和学科专业建设，促进中医药教育创新发展。

本套教材建设过程中，教材办聘请中医学、中药学、针灸推拿学三个专业的权威专家组成编审专家组，参与主编确定，提出指导意见，审查编写质量。特别是对核心示范教材建设加强了组织管理，成立了专门评价专家组，全程指导教材建设，确保教材质量。

本套教材具有以下特点：

1.坚持立德树人，融入课程思政内容

将党的二十大精神进教材，把立德树人贯穿教材建设全过程、各方面，体现课程思政建设新要求，发挥中医药文化育人优势，促进中医药人文教育与专业教育有机融合，指导学生树立正确世界观、人生观、价值观，帮助学生立大志、明大德、成大才、担大任，坚定信念信心，努力成为堪当民族复兴重任的时代新人。

2.优化知识结构，强化中医思维培养

在"十三五"规划教材知识架构基础上，进一步整合优化学科知识结构体系，减少不同学科教材间相同知识内容交叉重复，增强教材知识结构的系统性、完整性。强化中医思维培养，突出中医思维在教材编写中的主导作用，注重中医经典内容编写，在《内经》《伤寒论》等经典课程中更加突出重点，同时更加强化经典与临床的融合，增强中医经典的临床运用，帮助学生筑牢中医经典基础，逐步形成中医思维。

3.突出"三基五性",注重内容严谨准确

坚持"以本为本",更加突出教材的"三基五性",即基本知识、基本理论、基本技能,思想性、科学性、先进性、启发性、适用性。注重名词术语统一,概念准确,表述科学严谨,知识点结合完备,内容精炼完整。教材编写综合考虑学科的分化、交叉,既充分体现不同学科自身特点,又注意各学科之间的有机衔接;注重理论与临床实践结合,与医师规范化培训、医师资格考试接轨。

4.强化精品意识,建设行业示范教材

遴选行业权威专家,吸纳一线优秀教师,组建经验丰富、专业精湛、治学严谨、作风扎实的高水平编写团队,将精品意识和质量意识贯穿教材建设始终,严格编审把关,确保教材编写质量。特别是对32门核心示范教材建设,更加强调知识体系架构建设,紧密结合国家精品课程、一流学科、一流专业建设,提高编写标准和要求,着力推出一批高质量的核心示范教材。

5.加强数字化建设,丰富拓展教材内容

为适应新型出版业态,充分借助现代信息技术,在纸质教材基础上,强化数字化教材开发建设,对全国中医药行业教育云平台"医开讲"进行了升级改造,融入了更多更实用的数字化教学素材,如精品视频、复习思考题、AR/VR等,对纸质教材内容进行拓展和延伸,更好地服务教师线上教学和学生线下自主学习,满足中医药教育教学需要。

本套教材的建设,凝聚了全国中医药行业高等教育工作者的集体智慧,体现了中医药行业齐心协力、求真务实、精益求精的工作作风,谨此向有关单位和个人致以衷心的感谢!

尽管所有组织者与编写者竭尽心智,精益求精,本套教材仍有进一步提升空间,敬请广大师生提出宝贵意见和建议,以便不断修订完善。

国家中医药管理局教材办公室

中国中医药出版社有限公司

2023 年 6 月

编写说明

　　全国中医药行业高等教育"十四五"规划教材《护理专业英语》的编写是根据《中共中央 国务院关于促进中医药传承创新发展的意见》《国务院办公厅关于加快医学教育创新发展的指导意见》和《教育部 国家卫生健康委 国家中医药管理局关于深化医教协同进一步推动中医药教育改革与高质量发展的实施意见》的精神，在国家中医药管理局教材办公室宏观指导下，以全面提高中医药人才的培养质量、积极与医疗卫生实践接轨、为临床服务为目标，依据中医药行业人才培养规律和实际需求而完成。

　　作为护理学专业本科教材，《护理专业英语》的编写严格按照全国中医药行业高等教育护理学专业培养方案对专业英语教学的要求进行选材、设计，注意突出趣味性、专业性、实用性和系统性，力求融传授知识、培养技能、提高素质为一体，重视培养学生的评判性思维及终生学习的能力。主要内容是根据护理工作中经常遇到的情况，设置情景对话、专业文章和阅读材料，使学生了解西方国家护理文化及护理理念，掌握护理实践中所需的护理英语词汇、医患沟通交流技巧等，旨在提高学生的专业英语水平和运用能力。教材内容同时融入了思政元素，以提高学生的思政水平。另外，设置了一个中医护理英语的单元，突出中医护理特色，弘扬中医传统文化。

　　教材共设置 15 个单元，每单元为一个护理主题，包含听说训练、阅读两个板块，后附习题。以患者就诊、入院、住院、出院到家庭和社区为主线，内容涵盖了临床护理实践、护理理论、护理文化和伦理等与护理工作密切相关的知识和技能。在教学内容设置上，注重培养学生听、说、读、写、译的能力。教材还设有附录，包括习题答案、词汇表、视音频脚本、常用医学词根和词缀、常用药物、参考文献等内容。其中，视音频脚本文字忠实于原版素材。

　　本教材编写分工如下：第 1 单元由易平编写，第 2 单元由解东编写，第 3 单元由周芬编写，第 4 单元由周恩、吉彬彬编写，第 5 单元由周云仙编写，第 6 单元由安雪梅编写，第 7 单元由袁娟、李艳微编写，第 8 单元由潘兰霞编写，第 9 单元由叶丽萍、刘芃汐编写，第 10 单元由李绵利编写，第 11 单元由谷岩梅、刘红霞编写，第 12 单元由张姮编写，第 13 单元由余朝琴、刘娅编写，第 14 单元由陈战编写，第 15 单元由贾瑞敏编写，最后由刘红霞和刘娅统稿。

　　本教材融合出版数字化工作由刘红霞和刘娅负责，编委会全体人员参与。教材精品MOOC 由成都中医药大学监制，梁静负责编辑录制。

　　本教材所配套的教学视频由美国 Indiana University Kokomo School of Nursing, St, Joseph Hospital and Howard Regional Health System 共同参与录制，根据教材所提供的情景，录制了

美国医院的真实护理场景，并给予实例讲解什么是好的和不好的护理实践。通过观看视频，学生能够学习标准的美式口语、了解美国的医院情况和护理情况。

《护理专业英语》编委会

2021 年 4 月

目　录

扫一扫，查阅本章数字资源，含 PPT、音视频、图片等

After studying this unit, you are required to:

- **summarize the definitions and the nature of nursing**
- **master the basic knowledge of nursing practice in China**
- **explain the three models for nursing and their respective advantages and disadvantages**

Part Ⅰ Listening & Speaking

Task 1 Listening

Listen to the audio and discuss the following questions in pairs.

1) Why do not most people think nurses' work in "nursing home" is promising?

2) What is the challenge for a "nursing home" nurse?

3) What will the speaker still remember when she looks back on her career?

Task 2 Dialogue

In pairs, practice the following dialogue and remember the useful words and expressions.

ADVISING A NEW COLLEGE NURSING STUDENT

(F: Nursing Faculty   S: Nursing Student)

S: Good morning, Professor Li. My name is Wang Fang, I am a freshman and your advisee. May I ask you some questions?

F: Great! Nice to meet you, Wang Fang. Come in please and take a seat.

S: I am a new nursing student and I want to know more about nursing. Would you please tell about its history?

F: Florence Nightingale is known as the founder of modern nursing. She made outstanding contributions to the wounded soldiers during the Crimean War. She also established a training program for nurses at St. Thomas Hospital in London, the first formal nursing program in the world. She had many publications—her book, *Notes on Nursing: What It Is and What It Is Not*, has been described as one of the seminal works of the modern world. The Nightingale Pledge, taken by new nurses, was named in her honor, and the annual International Nurses Day is celebrated on her birthday.

S: Great, then, what is the fundamental difference between nursing and medicine?

F: That is a good question. As you probably know, both medicine and nursing are health professions, but they are two different branches of health science. Medicine focuses on providing effective treatments to cure the diseases, while nursing pays more attention to caring for a client's physio-psycho-social responses related to certain diseases.

S: What are the major roles and functions of a registered nurse?

F: Historically, the caregiver is the principal role of a nurse. As nursing has evolved, the roles and functions of a nurse have been expanded. In addition to performing as a caregiver, a nurse may work as a communicator, educator, client advocate, counselor, leader, manager, researcher, and so on.

S: That's very inspiring! Now, my last question, what are the core courses for students in the baccalaureate nursing program?

F: Well, courses vary from school to school. In general, the core courses include, but are not limited to, fundamentals of nursing, medical-surgical nursing, pediatric nursing, obstetrical and gynecological nursing, community nursing, geriatric nursing, nursing research, nursing education, and nursing management.

S: That's really very informative. I feel like I know more about nursing now!

F: I am very pleased that you found this information helpful. Please do not hesitate to contact me if you have further questions or other needs! See you then.

S: Thank you, Professor Li. See you.

Part Ⅱ Reading

Reading Guidance

What is nursing? What are the unique functions of nursing? As a future nurse, you may have these questions in mind. In this unit, we are going to explore the nature of nursing and different perspectives about nursing. Especially, we will introduce the practice of nursing in China, which is related to clinical nursing, community-based health care, nursing education, nursing management and nursing research. Then you will know the advantages and disadvantages of the functional nursing, team nursing and primary nursing.

Before Class

Please think carefully about these questions and discuss with your classmates.

- **What do you think is the definition of nursing?**

- **What is the nature of nursing?**

- **What do you think about the practice of nursing in China?**

TEXT A   Modern Views on Nursing

The Definitions of Nursing

Nursing has been defined differently in the literature depending on the historical era. The most influential definitions about nursing were introduced by the following nursing scholars and nursing organizations.

Florence Nightingale, the founder of modern nursing, is probably the first one to formally define nursing. In the well-known publication *Notes on Nursing: What It Is and What It Is Not*, Nightingale wrote, "Nature alone cures … and what nursing has to do is to put the patient in the best condition for nature to act upon him. Nursing ought to signify the proper use of fresh air, light, warmth, cleanliness, quiet, and the proper selection of administration of diet—all at the expense of vital power of the patient. Nursing creates the environment most conducive to body's reparative processes".

The best known definition of nursing is probably the one developed by Virginia Henderson who wrote, "the unique function of the nurse is to assist the individual, sick or well, in the performance of those activities contributing to health or its recovery (or to peaceful death) that he would perform unaided if he had the necessary strength, will or knowledge". This definition was adopted by the International Council of Nurses (ICN) in 1960 and is still the most widely and internationally used definition of nursing.

Another well-known definition of nursing was developed by the American Nurses Association (ANA), which stated that "nursing is the protection, promotion, and optimization of health and abilities; prevention of illness and injury; alleviation of suffering through the diagnosis and treatment of human responses; and advocacy in health care for individuals, families, communities, and populations".

In 2002, ICN offers a definition of nursing similar to that of ANA. According to the ICN, "nursing encompasses autonomous and collaborative care of individuals of all ages, families, groups and communities, sick or well and in all settings. Nursing includes the promotion of health, prevention of illness, and the care of ill, disabled and dying people. Advocacy, promotion of a safe environment, research, participation in shaping health policy and in patient and health systems management, and education are also key nursing roles".

The Nature of Nursing

Nursing has been recognized as both an art and a science. Nursing has also been considered a young profession, a practice discipline.

Nursing as an Art. When we talk about the art of nursing, we emphasize the intuitive, creative, and imaginative aspect of nursing. As Donahue wrote, "Nursing is not merely a technique but a process that incorporates the elements of soul, mind, and imagination. Its very essence lies in the creative imagination, the sensitive spirit, and the intelligent understanding that provide the very foundation for effective nursing care".

Art is also the reflection of feelings and perceptions. Because the core and essence of nursing is caring and personal interaction, the art of nursing finds expression in many ways: for example, in a nurse's sensitivity and perception of a client's thoughts and feelings and the nurse's expression of thoughts and feelings to the client.

Traditional nursing as art was predominate in the first half of the 20th century when nursing was largely the care of the ill in the hospital. Nursing was primarily the art of caring, based on intuition and skill training rather than on science. As nursing has continued to evolve as a profession, the scientific aspect of nursing has been gradually recognized without devaluing the art of nursing.

Nursing as a Science. Science is concerned with causality (cause and effect). Parse defines science as the "theoretical explanation of the subject of inquiry and the methodological process of sustaining knowledge in a discipline". Science is both a process and product. As a process, science is characterized by systematic inquiry that relies heavily on empirical observations of the natural world. As a product, it has been defined as empirical knowledge that is grounded and tested in experience. Science can be classified as pure or basic science, natural science, human or social science, and applied or practical science.

In general, nursing science refers to the system of relationships of human responses in health and illness addressing biologic, behavioral, social, and cultural domains. Florence Nightingale identified nursing as a scientific discipline separated from medicine, emphasizing the idea of creating freestanding nursing schools where nurses (rather than doctors) assumed responsibility for nursing education. The integration of science and art in nursing, consequently, has been facilitated.

The shift of nursing education from hospitals to universities has advanced the science of nursing. University-based nursing education provides nurses the educational foundation necessary to make scientific applications in nursing practice. Graduate nursing education prepares nurses with advanced research and critical thinking skills, and a working knowledge of theories from other scientific disciplines, which contribute to further advancements in nursing science.

Nursing as a Profession. In the past, there has been considerable discussion about whether nursing is a profession or an occupation. It is necessary to differentiate these two terms here. An occupation is a job or a career, whereas a profession is a learned vocation or occupation that has a status of superiority within a division of work. All professions are occupations, but not all occupations are professions.

To answer whether nursing is a profession, we need to know the characteristics of a profession. In general, all professions have the following features:

1) A body of knowledge on which skills and services are based

2) Ability to deliver a unique service to society

3) Education that is standardized and based in colleges and universities

4) Control of standards for practice through professional registration and licensing

5) Responsibility and accountability of members for their own actions

6) Career commitment by members

7) Autonomy

Traditionally, nursing was viewed as an occupation rather than a profession. Nursing has had difficulty being deemed a profession because the services provided by nurses have been perceived as an extension of those offered by wives and mothers. Additionally, historically nursing has been seen as subservient to medicine, and nurses have delayed identifying their unique body of knowledge. Furthermore, autonomy in practice is in question because nursing is still dependent on medicine to direct some of its practice.

However, many of the characteristics of a profession can be observed in modern nursing. Nurses provide services to meet health care needs for clients at different points in the health-illness continuum. There is a growing knowledge base, authority over education, a code of ethics, and registration requirements for practice. Hence, many nurses believe that nursing is an aspiring, evolving profession.

New Words

signify ['sɪgnɪfaɪ] *vt.*	表示；意味；预示
optimization [ˌɒptɪmaɪ'zeɪʃən] *n.*	最佳化，最优化
alleviation [əˌliːvi'eɪʃn] *n.*	减轻，缓解；镇痛剂
advocacy ['ædvəkəsɪ] *n.*	主张；拥护；辩护
encompass [ɪn'kʌmpəs] *vt.*	包含；包围，环绕
collaborative [kə'læbəretɪv] *adj.*	合作的，协作的
perception [pə'sepʃn] *n.*	知觉；看法；洞察力
intuition [ˌɪntju'ɪʃn] *n.*	直觉
empirical [ɪm'pɪrɪkl] *adj.*	经验主义的，完全根据经验的
accountability [əˌkaʊntə'bɪləti] *n.*	有义务；有责任
autonomy [ɔː'tɒnəmi] *n.*	自治，自治权
subservient [səb'sɜːvɪənt] *adj.*	屈从的
authority [ɔː'θɒrəti] *n.*	权威；权力；当局
ethics ['eθɪks] *n.*	伦理学；伦理观；道德标准

TEXT B   Contemporary Professional Nursing

Dimensions of Nursing Practice

Currently in China, the practice of nursing is related to the following aspects or dimensions:

Clinical nursing. In clinical nursing, nurses generally practice in hospitals. Clients are the recipients of clinical nursing. Clinical nursing practice is implemented based on nursing science and related disciplinary theories, knowledge and skills. Evidence-based nursing, holistic nursing ideas and perspectives affect the practice of clinical nursing. Clinical nursing practice includes basic nursing, specialty nursing and diagnostic and treatment nursing skills.

Community-based health care. Community-based health care, as the term indicates, is nursing care directed toward a specific population or group within the community. In community-based health care, or more specifically, community nursing, nurses work in communities. Nurses use clinical nursing knowledge and skills to provide services aiming at health promotion, health maintenance and illness prevention.

Nursing education. Nursing education refers to formal learning and training in the science of nursing. It involves the application of educational theories in training nursing students with the necessary knowledge and skills to practice nursing. The aim of nursing education is to develop nursing students morally, psychologically, intellectually and aesthetically.

Nursing management. Nursing management is performing the leadership function of governance and decision-making within the nurse-related health care organizations. It includes processes common to all management like planning, organizing, staffing, directing and controlling. The major components of nursing management include the person (namely, nurses), fiscal and human resources, equipment and facilities, time, and information. The aim of nursing management is to ensure the services provided by nurses are appropriate, timely, safe, and effective in order to meet the clients' health care needs.

Nursing research. Nursing research is "the systematic, rigorous, logical investigation that aims to answer questions about nursing phenomena". Nursing research requires the researcher to follow the steps of the scientific processes. There are two types of research, quantitative and qualitative. Nursing research generates a specialized scientific knowledge base that empowers the nursing profession to anticipate and meet constantly shifting challenges and to maintain social relevance.

Models of nursing care delivery

Nursing care delivery models provide a framework to organize the work of caring for patients. There are basically three methods for assigning nurses to the day-to-day care of patients in the hospital. They are functional nursing, team nursing, and primary nursing.

Functional nursing. Functional nursing divides nursing work into functional units that are then assigned to one of the team members. In this model, each care provider is responsible for specific duties or tasks. Hence, in functional nursing, the emphasis is on the task. The advantages of utilizing functional nursing include: (1) care can be delivered to a large number of patients in a short time; and (2) auxiliary health workers with certain nursing skills can be used when there is a shortage of registered nurses (RNs). The disadvantages of this care delivery model are obvious, the care of the patient is fragmented; patients are usually not treated as individuals or given comprehensive care.

Team nursing. Team nursing is a care delivery model that assigns staff to teams that are then responsible for a group of patients. A unit is divided into two or more teams, each led by a registered nurse. The team leader supervises and coordinates all of the care provided by those on the team. Care is divided into the simplest components and then assigned to the care provider with the appropriate level of skills. The advantages of adopting team nursing include: (1) high-quality comprehensive care can be provided despite a relatively high proportion of ancillary staff on the team; (2) each member of the team is able to participate in decision making and problem solving; (3) each team member is able to contribute his/her own special skills in caring for the patient; and (4) team nursing has demonstrated improved patient satisfaction; and (5) an RN directs and evaluates the care of all patients. However, there are disadvantages: communication is complex within the team, a team may not always work effectively together; the team leader may not have the leadership skills required to effectively direct the team; and shared responsibility and accountability can cause confusion and lack of accountability.

Primary nursing. Primary nursing is a care delivery model which emphasizes continuity of care by having one nurse (called the primary nurse) organize complete care for a small group of inpatients within a nursing unit of a hospital. The primary nurse is responsible for planning and evaluating the care delivered to the assigned patients 24 hours a day. Associate nurses care for the patient when the primary nurse is not working. The advantages of this model include: (1) development of a trusting relationship between the patient, family and primary nurse; (2) encouragement of a holistic approach to care, facilitation of continuity of care; (3) definition of the accountability and responsibility of the nurse in developing a plan of care with the patient and family; and (4) authority for clinical decision making is given to the nurse at the bedside. However, the cost is high due to the requirement of a higher RN skill mix. Additionally, nurses report stress, role overload, and role ambiguity.

New Words

dimension [daɪ'menʃn; dɪ'menʃn] *n.*	方面；［数］维；尺寸
implement ['ɪmplɪm(ə)nt] *vt.*	实施，执行；使生效
holistic [hə'lɪstɪk] *adj.*	整体的；全盘的
perspective [pə'spektɪv] *n.*	观点，视角；远景
aesthetically [iːs'θetɪkli; es'θetɪkli] a*dv.*	审美地；美学观点上地
component [kəm'pəʊnənt] *n.*	成分；组件
fiscal ['fɪskl] *adj.*	会计的，财政的
empower [ɪm'paʊə(r)] *vt.*	授权，允许；使能够
auxiliary [ɔːg'zɪliəri] *adj.*	辅助的；副的；附加的
ambiguity [ˌæmbɪ'gjuːəti] *n.*	含糊；不明确；模棱两可的话

FOLLOW–UP ACTIVITIES

Translation

A. Translate the following sentences into Chinese.

1. Nursing includes the promotion of health, prevention of illness, and the care of ill, disabled and dying people.

_____

_____

2. Nursing is not merely a technique but a process that incorporates the elements of soul, mind, and imagination.

_____

_____

3. In general, nursing science refers to the system of relationships of human responses in health and illness addressing biologic, behavioral, social, and cultural domains.

_____

_____

4. The unique function of the nurse is to assist the individual, sick or well, in the performance of those activities contributing to health or its recovery (or to peaceful death) that he would perform unaided if he had the necessary strength, will or knowledge.

_____

_____

B. Translate the following sentences into English.

1. 以人为中心的护理强调对整个人的护理，即对身体、思想和精神的护理。

_____

_____

2. 自我意识和自我保健是综合护理重要的核心实施部分。

_____

_____

3. 帮助患者是护士的天职。在你的内心，应该有一种欲望和动力驱使你为提高别人的生命质量做些事情。

_____

_____

4. 护理理论是对护理实践的系统的抽象性概括。其目的在于描述、解释、预测或控制护理行为以实现一定的护理目标。

_____

_____

Admitting and Discharging a Patient

扫一扫，查阅本章数字资源，含PPT、音视频、图片等

After studying this unit, you are required to:

● master the basic knowledge of nursing in the aspect of nurse-patient relationship

● be able to admit and discharge a foreign patient in English

Part Ⅰ Listening & Speaking

Task 1 Listening

1. Watch the video and discuss the following questions in pairs.

1) What do you think the nurse is doing?

2) What information might you need to collect in this situation?

3) Why might this information be important?

4) What strategies have you found useful when greeting a patient for the first time?

2. Dawn, the ward nurse, is admitting Mrs. Johns. Listen to the conversation and answer the following questions.

1) Is Mrs. Johns mobile?

2) Has she been sick?

3) Why is Mrs. Johns in hospital?

4) What were the oxygen saturations of Mrs. Johns on admission?

5) What were her vital signs at 11∶30 a.m.?

6) Did Dr. Brown order any medication for her headache?

3. Role-Play

Prepare nurse-patient interviews. Student A, the nurse, looks at the Patient Admission Form and thinks about the questions you will be asked to complete it. Student B, the patient, tries to answer those questions.

PATIENT ADMISSION FORM

Full Name	
Address	
DOB (Date of Birth)	
Past medical history	
Reason for admission	
Chief complaint	
Allergies	

4. Dialogue Making

Make a dialogue in which the nurse is introducing the ward routines to the patient. The following may serve as the guidelines.

Bed No.	Bed 2, Room 602
Ward	the medical ward
Bed nurse	Zhang Ping
Doctor in charge	Dr. Liu
Personal articles	kept in the admission office or ...
Personal care items	toothpaste, toothbrush, slippers, comb ...
A nurse-call system	the panel on the head of the bed
Ward rules	visiting hours, meal time, types of meal served, location of bathroom and toilet
The patient's needs	any special needs
Ward round and treatment time	8 a.m.

Task 2 Dialogue

In pairs, practice the following dialogue and remember the useful words and expressions.

DISCHARGING A PATIENT

Discharging plan starts after the patient is admitted to the hospital. Health education is one of the most important aspects of discharge planning. Before discharging a patient home or to other settings, it's crucial to assess patient's self-care ability and to carry out the health education.

(N: Nurse　　P: Patient)

N: Hello, Mr. Little. I am glad to know that you will go home in a couple of days. In order to help you prepare for this, I need to know more about your life at home if you don't mind.

P: Of course I don't mind.

N: Ok. I have a discharge checklist in hand. I want to make sure you will be looked after by someone at home as needed. I will also contact the GP (general practitioner) to let him/her know what happened to you during your hospital stay.

P: Ok, that is very kind of you.

N: I have your address here, is it a flat with easy access, I mean that the wheelchair can move through easily?

P: Yes, I have used my wheelchair for years. The stairs got sorted out already.

N: Great! So only the Zimmer frame is new to you? I will ask the social worker to complete a safety evaluation in your flat before your discharge date so that any potential risk will be removed.

P: That is very considerate, I appreciate it.

N: My pleasure. You will continue to take some medications and vitamins after discharge. I shall arrange for the district nurse to check with you each week about your medication, to make sure that you take the right medication at the right time and in the right amount.

P: Yeah, I think that will be very helpful.

N: Is there anything else you think you may need help with while you are at home by yourself?

P: Hmm... I could manage cooking for myself. But... but I may need some help with shopping, as I cannot lift heavy items, such as milk and juice.

N: Ok. How often do you go to the grocery?

P: Once a week.

N: Sure. I will arrange social workers to do that for you, your job is to give a shopping list to them.

P: No problem.

N: Your follow-up appointment with Dr. White has been made for 10 a.m. Wednesday, November 11th at the out-patient department, 2nd floor Jeffery Wing, St. Mary's hospital. If you cannot make the appointment, please call the number on the bottom of the appointment card and reschedule.

P: I certainly will.

N: Thank you. I am going to prepare some documents for you and your GP. Meanwhile, if you need any other assistance, please do not hesitate to let me know.

P: I will, thanks a lot.

N: My pleasure.

Part II Reading

Reading Guidance

Patient may need to know about the different departments and categories of professionals working in the hospital. Being a member of the medical staff, we must be familiar with the organization structure, function, medical staff, and management of a hospital. In this part, we will focus on the process of admitting patients into the unit. A nurse should be able to deal with the irrational use of medications and some common disorders, such as acute interstitial nephritis (AIN) caused by side effects of certain drugs.

Before Class
Please think carefully about these questions and discuss with your classmates.

● **What departments does a general hospital consist of?**

● **What are the differences between the in-patient and out-patient departments?**

● **Who are involved in health care practice in clinical settings?**

● **What are the characteristics of various professionals?**

TEXT A   Hospital

A hospital is a health care institution providing patient treatment by specialized staff using special equipment. Hospitals often, but not always, provide for inpatient care or longer term patient stays.

Organization Structure of a Hospital

Hospitals may be divided into general hospitals and specialty hospitals. A general hospital that is set up to deal with many kinds of diseases and injuries may consist of such departments as medical, surgical, pediatric, obstetric and gynecological, dental, skin, and traditional Chinese medicine, etc. Types of specialized hospitals include trauma centers, rehabilitation hospitals, children's hospitals, seniors (geriatric) hospitals, and hospitals for dealing with specific medical needs such as psychiatric problems, and certain disease categories such as cardiac, oncological, or orthopedic.

Function of a Hospital

Hospital functions have evolved from providing care for the sick to providing preventive, promotive, curative and rehabilitative services. Hospitals vary widely in the services they offer and therefore, in the departments they contain. Hospitals mainly consist of two major departments: the out-patient department and the in-patient department. They may have acute services such as an emergency department or specialist trauma centre, burn unit, surgery, or urgent care. There are consulting rooms in the out-patient department. An out-patient is a patient who is not hospitalized for more than 24 hours but who visits a hospital, clinic, or associated facility for diagnosis or treatment. Treatment provided in this fashion is called ambulatory care.

There are wards and intensive care units in the in-patient department. An in-patient, is "admitted" to the hospital and stays overnight or for an indeterminate time, usually several days or weeks (though some cases, like coma patients, have been in hospitals for years). Treatment provided in this fashion is called in-patient care. The admission to the hospital involves the creation of an admission note. Leaving the hospital is officially termed discharge, and requires a corresponding discharge note.

A hospital has many sections or parts, including a registration office, a dispensary (pharmacy), laboratory, blood bank, central supply room, operating rooms, and radiology (X-ray and computerized tomography) rooms.

Medical Staff

An individual health care practitioner (also known as a health worker) may be a health care professional, allied health professional, or another person trained and knowledgeable in medicine, nursing or other allied health professions. Health care practitioners include physicians, surgeons, dentists, nurses, midwives, pharmacists, dietitians, therapists, psychologists, clinical officers, emergency medical technicians, medical laboratory scientists, and radiographers, etc. A surgical practitioner is a health worker who specializes in the planning and delivery of a patient's perioperative care during the anesthetic, surgical and recovery stages. They may include general and specialist surgeons, anesthesiologists, nurse anesthetists, surgical nurses, and others. A maternal and newborn health practitioner is a health worker who deals with the care of women and their children before, during and after pregnancy and childbirth. These include obstetricians, midwives, nurse practitioners, and others. A mental health practitioner is a health worker who offers services for the purpose of improving an individual's mental health or treating mental illness. These include psychiatrists, clinical psychologists, mental health practitioners, and others. A geriatric care practitioner plans and coordinates the care of the elderly and/or disabled to promote their health, improve their quality of life, and maintain their independence as long as possible. They include geriatricians, geriatric nurses, geriatric aides, and others who focus on the health and psychological care needs of older adults.

Management System

All medical staff work under the director or superintendent of a hospital. Under the superintendent we have the head of each department, such as the head of the department of medical administration, the head of the nursing department, the head of the out-patient department, the head of the surgical department, the head of the medical department, etc. Under the heads of departments we have other medical staff. For example, under the head of medical department, we may have physicians in charge, resident physicians, interns, head nurses and nurses, etc. All medical staff give their services for the patients.

New Words

institution [ˌɪnstɪˈtuːʃən] *n.*	公共机构，协会，慈善机构
specialize [ˈspeʃəlaɪz] *v.*	专业化，专门化
staff [stɑːf] *n.*	医务人员，工作人员
pediatric [ˌpidɪˈætrɪk] *adj.*	儿科的
obstetric [əbˈstetrɪk] *adj.*	产科（学）的
gynecological [ˌɡaɪnɪkəˈlɒdʒɪkəl] *adj.*	妇科（学）的
rehabilitation [ˌriːəˌbɪlɪˈteɪʃn] *n.*	康复（医学）
geriatric [ˌdʒerɪˈætrɪk] *adj.*	老年医学的
oncological [ɑnkəˈlɒdʒikl] *n.*	肿瘤学
orthopedic [ˌɔːθəˈpiːdɪk] *adj.*	整形外科的
emergency [ɪˈmɜːdʒənsi] *n.*	急诊，意外
ambulatory [ˈæmbjələtəri] *adj.*	移动的，走动的
dispensary [dɪˈspensəri] *n.*	药房，诊疗所
practitioner [prækˈtɪʃənə(r)] *n.*	开业医生，从业者
physician [fɪˈzɪʃn] *n.*	医师，内科医师
surgeon [ˈsɜːdʒən] *n.*	外科医生
dentist [ˈdentɪst] *n.*	牙科医生
midwife [ˈmɪdwaɪf] *n.*	助产士
pharmacist [ˈfɑːməsɪst] *n.*	药剂师
dietitian [ˌdaɪəˈtɪʃn] *n.*	营养师
therapist [ˈθerəpɪst] *n.*	治疗师
radiographer [ˌreɪdɪˈɑɡrəfə˞] *n.*	放射科技师
psychiatrist [saɪˈkaɪətrɪst] *n.*	精神病专家，精神病医师
psychologist [saɪˈkɒlədʒɪst] *n.*	心理学家
superintendent [ˌsupərɪnˈtendənt] *n.*	院长，负责人
intern [ˈɪntɜːn] *n.*	实习医师

TEXT B   Interstitial Nephritis

Interstitial nephritis is a kidney disorder in which the spaces between the kidney tubules become swollen (inflamed). This can cause problems with the way the kidneys work. Interstitial nephritis may be temporary (acute), or it may be long-lasting (chronic) and get worse over time.

Causes

The acute form of interstitial nephritis is most often caused by side effects of certain drugs. Acute interstitial nephritis (AIN) is an important cause of acute kidney injury that has experienced significant epidemiological and clinical changes in the last years. Drug-induced AIN continues to be the commonest type, but it requires a careful differential diagnosis to distinguish it from other entities. New diagnostic tests and biomarkers, as well as prospective therapeutic studies are needed to improve AIN diagnosis and management.

The following can cause interstitial nephritis:

● Allergic reaction to a drug (acute interstitial allergic nephritis).

● Autoimmune disorders such as anti-tubular basement membrane disease, Kawasaki's disease, Sjogren syndrome, systemic lupus erythematosus, or Wegener's granulomatosis.

● Infections.

● Long-term use of medications such as acetaminophen (Tylenol), aspirin, and nonsteroidal anti-inflammatory drugs (NSAIDS). This is called analgesic nephropathy.

● Side effect of certain antibiotics (including penicillin, ampicillin, methicillin, sulfonamide medications, and others).

● Side effect of other medications such as furosemide, thiazide diuretics, omeprazole, triamterene, and allopurinol.

● Too little potassium in the blood.

● Too much calcium or uric acid in the blood.

Symptoms

Interstitial nephritis can cause mild to severe kidney problems, including acute kidney failure. In about half of the cases, people will have decreased urine output and other signs of acute kidney failure.

Symptoms of this condition may include:

● Blood in the urine.

● Fever.

● Increased or decreased urine output.

● Mental status changes (drowsiness, confusion, coma).

● Nausea, vomiting.

● Rash.

● Swelling of the body, any area.

● Weight gain (from retaining fluid).

Exams and Tests

The health care provider will perform a physical exam. This may reveal abnormal lung or heart sounds, high blood pressure, or fluid in the lungs (pulmonary edema). Common tests include arterial blood gases, blood chemistry, blood urea nitrogen (BUN) and blood creatinine levels, complete blood count, kidney biopsy, kidney ultrasound and urinalysis.

Treatment

Treatment depends on the cause of the problem. Avoiding medications that lead to this condition may relieve symptoms quickly. Limiting salt and fluid in the diet can improve swelling and high blood pressure. Limiting protein in the diet can help control the buildup of waste products in the blood (azotemia) that can lead to symptoms of acute kidney failure. If dialysis is necessary, it usually is required for only a short time. Corticosteroids or stronger anti-inflammatory medications such as cyclophosphamide can sometimes be helpful.

Outlook (Prognosis)

Most often, interstitial nephritis is a short-term disorder. In rare cases, it can cause permanent damage, including chronic kidney failure. Acute interstitial nephritis may be more severe and more likely to lead to long-term or permanent kidney damage in elderly people.

Possible Complications

Metabolic acidosis can occur because the kidneys are not able to remove enough acid. The disorder can lead to acute or chronic kidney failure or end-stage kidney disease.

When to Contact a Medical Professional

Call your health care provider if you have symptoms of interstitial nephritis. Call your health care provider if you get new symptoms, especially if you are less alert or have a decrease in urine output.

Prevention

In many cases, the disorder can't be prevented. Avoiding or reducing your use of medications that can cause this condition can help reduce your risk. The reasons for the irrational use of drugs or combined products included easy availability without prescription; ignorance of harmful effects; misleading advertisements; and attractive incentives for marketing and/or prescribing. The public should be educated about the harmful effects of drugs, and especially of self-medication. More emphasis is needed on preventative aspects of health rather than curative ones. Availability of drug information to all practitioners from independent sources and periodic audit of prescriptions may help to curb misuse of drugs. Medical associations should urge the government to ban harmful drugs and irrational combinations, and request a secure supply of essential drugs.

New Words

interstitial [ˌɪntə'stɪʃl] *adj.*	间质的；空隙的
nephritis [nɪ'fraɪtɪs] *n.*	肾炎
disorder [dɪs'ɔːdə(r)] *n.*	（身体、精神的）失调；不适
swollen ['swəʊlən] *adj.*	肿胀的；浮肿的
epidemiological [ˌepɪˌdiːmiə'lɒdʒɪkl] *adj.*	流行病学的
erythematosus [ˌɛriˌθiː'mətəʊsəs] *n. adj.*	全身性红斑狼疮；红斑的
granulomatosis ['grænjuˌləʊmə'təʊsis] *n.*	［医］肉芽肿病
（复数 granulomatoses）	
potassium [pə'tæsɪəm] *n.*	［化学］钾
calcium ['kælsɪəm] *n.*	［化学］钙
analgesic [ˌænəl'dʒiːzɪk] *adj. n.*	止痛的；止痛剂；［药］镇痛剂
nephropathy [nə'frɒpəθi] *n.*	［泌尿］肾病
biopsy ['baɪɒpsi] *n.*	活体组织检查
creatinine [krɪ'ætɪniːn] *n.*	［生化］肌酸酐
dialysis [ˌdaɪ'æləsɪs] *n.*	透析
prognosis [prɒg'nəʊsɪs] *n.*	预后；预知
complication [ˌkɒmplɪ'keɪʃn] *n.*	并发症

FOLLOW–UP ACTIVITIES

Translation

A. Translate the following sentences into Chinese.

1. Hospitals vary widely in the services they offer and therefore, in the departments they contain. However, most hospitals consist of two major departments: the out-patient department and the in-patient department.

_____

_____

2. An out-patient is a patient who is not hospitalized for more than 24 hours but who visits a hospital, clinic, or associated facility for diagnosis or treatment. Treatment provided in this fashion is called ambulatory care.

_____

_____

3. The admission to the hospital involves the creation of an admission note. Leaving the hospital is officially termed discharge, and requires a corresponding discharge note.

_____

_____

4. Drug-induced AIN (acute interstitial nephritis) continues to be the commonest type, but it requires a careful differential diagnosis to distinguish it from other entities.

_____

_____

B. Translate the following paragraphs into English.

1. 医疗卫生服务执业者包括内科医生、外科医生、牙科医生、护士、药剂师、营养师、治疗师、心理医生、临床行政人员、急诊医疗技师、临床检验专家（技师）和放射科技师等。

_____

_____

2. 医院由很多部门组成，包括挂号室、药房、检验科、血库、中心供应室、手术室和放射科（X线和计算机横断面扫描）。

_____

_____

3. 避免服用导致急性间质性肾炎的药物可能很快减轻症状。限制饮食中的盐和液体的摄入能改善水肿和高血压。

_____

_____

4. 老年人患有急性间质性肾炎可能会更严重，也更可能引起长期或永久的肾功能损伤。

_____

_____

Unit Three
Health Assessment

扫一扫，查阅本章数字资源，含PPT、音视频、图片等

After studying this unit, you are required to:

● **have mastered the basic knowledge of health assessment**

● **be able to assess a patient with respiratory disorder in English**

Part Ⅰ Listening & Speaking

Task 1 Video Watching

1. Watch the video and discuss the following questions in pairs.

1) Why does the nurse give a red bracelet to the patient?

2) What are the patient's main complaints?

3) How does the doctor build up the patient's confidence?

4) What strategies have you found useful when taking medical history from a patient?

2. Linda, the Ward Nurse, is admitting Miss Jones. Listen to the conversation and answer the following questions.

1) Why is Miss Jones in hospital?

2) Does she have any allergies?

3) Is Miss Jones a smoker?

4) What's the diagnosis of Miss Jones based on her chest X-ray?

5) How long would Miss Jones stay in CCPU?

3. Work in pairs and conduct a mock nurse-patient interview. Student A, the nurse, looks at the Patient Admission Form and thinks about the questions that need to be asked to complete it. Student B, the patient, tries to answer these questions.

PATIENT HEALTH HISTORY FORM

Full Name	
Gender	
Allergies	
Chief complaints	
Medication history	

4. Work in pairs and discuss how you might change your approach when taking health history

from the following patients.

1) A seven-year-old boy.

2) A pregnant woman.

Task 2 Dialogue

In pairs, practice the following dialogue and remember the useful words and expressions.

TAKING HEALTH HISTORY FROM A COPD PATIENT

(N: Nurse　　P: Patient)

N: First, please tell me the exact time when you started to experience breathing difficulty for the most recent episode.

P: Yesterday afternoon, about 2 p.m., I think. At that time I was going upstairs because the elevator in the building was not working.

N: So you became short of breath with exercise. How often do you feel short of breath?

P: Sometimes, but it was more frequent this week, three times already.

N: How long have you been feeling short of breath?

P: About one year. But this week it got worse, yesterday it lasted for about ten minutes, I guess.

N: How far can you walk, and how many steps can you climb before having to stop because of shortness of breath?

P: 200 meters, I think. Usually, the shortness of breath happens after I climb about 50 stairs, around 3 floors.

N: Do you cough?

P: Yes, every morning when I get up, I cough a lot.

N: How long have you been coughing? Is it getting worse?

P: About 5 years. It's getting worse these days.

N: Do you cough up mucus ? (nods "yes") You do. Ok, now tell me what color it is?

P: Yellow-green.

N: Have you ever coughed up blood?

P: Never.

N: Do you smoke?

P: I started smoking when I was 16 years old. I still remember I smoked at least 2 packs a day when I was 20. However, I quit smoking last year.

N: Great. Have you been exposed to airborne irritants, such as dust or chemicals, on the job?

P: I am a cleaner. I am exposed to dust every day.

…

Part Ⅱ Reading

Reading Guidance

As we all know, the first step of the nursing process is nursing assessment, in which a nurse

needs to take a comprehensive medical history from a patient. However, what should a nurse ask about? Why is the information in a health history so important? How do nurses take a health history from a patient with respiratory disorder? This text is going to provide answers to these questions.

Before Class

Please think carefully about these questions and discuss with your classmates.

- What are the contents of a health history?

- Why is age important for a patient with respiratory disorder?

- What are the three major respiratory symptoms?

TEXT A   Health Assessment on a Patient with Respiratory Disorder

When a patient with respiratory disorder is seen for the first time by the health care provider, the first requirement is that the baseline information be obtained (except in emergency situations when this data collection may occur simultaneously with life-saving procedures). The sequence and format of data collection about a patient may be varied, but the contents are usually the same. They are as follows:

Biographical Data

Biographical information includes the patient's name, address, age, gender, marital status, occupation, ethnic origins, etc. A quick review of the biographical data may identify actual or potential problems. How old is the patient? Respiratory structure and function change with age. For example, young children are more susceptible to respiratory infections because their airways are smaller and they have an immature immune system, but as people age, their forced expiratory volume decreases. Residence and occupation also have an impact on the respiratory system because a person's job or environment may harbor risk factors.

Current Health Status

The history of the current health concern or illness is the most important factor in helping the health care providers arrive at a diagnosis or determine the patient's needs. Information about the current health concern or illness helps in the selection of appropriate diagnostic tests and follow-up assessments.

Usually, begin with the patient's chief complaint (the issue that brings a patient to the health care provider). The three major respiratory symptoms to observe are dyspnea, cough, and chest pain. If you notice signs of respiratory distress, such as shortness of breath (SOB), confusion, or anxiety, postpone the detailed history and focus on the acute problem. Obtain a detailed history later, when the patient's condition improves, or get it from a secondary source such as a family member.

A patient with chronic respiratory disease often adapts to a compromised respiratory status. Therefore, compare the patient's present respiratory status with his or her status at previous examinations to evaluate the impact of the disease progression.

Symptom Analysis

Cough. Coughing is one of the most common respiratory complaints. The causes range from insignificant to life-threatening conditions. Coughing is a protective, reflexive mechanism that helps maintain a patent airway. It occurs in three phases: Deep inspiration that increases lung volume, closure of the glottis, and then muscular contraction forcing the sudden opening of the glottis, resulting in a cough. Cough receptors, located in the larynx, respiratory tree, pleura, acoustic duct, nose, sinuses, pharynx, stomach, and diaphragm respond to mechanical, inflammatory, or irritating stimuli.

Dyspnea. Dyspnea is a subjective sensation of breathing difficulty often described as SOB. It might be normal for a person with anxiety, but it may also signal underlying cardiopulmonary or neuromuscular problems or allergic reactions.

Chest pain. There are numerous chest pain assessment tools and here is a sample of them, CHEST, which can aid in the assessment of chest pain: C–commenced when; H–history/evidence of risk factors; E–extra/additional symptoms; S–stays/radiation; T–timing, how long has it lasted?

Related symptoms. Other symptoms associated with respiratory disease include edema and fatigue. Edema results from right-side congestive heart failure, a common complication of chronic obstructive lung disease. Usually, edema is located in the lower extremities or abdomen. Ask your patient, "Do you have swelling in your abdomen, legs, ankles, or feet?"

Hypoxia, increased energy expended for breathing, and associated cardiac involvement accompany long-standing lung disease and contribute to the development of fatigue. People adapt to fatigue by lowering their activity level, so they have more difficulty performing activities of daily living (ADLs). Changes in rest and sleep patterns may also be seen. Ask your patient, "Do you have enough energy to do your usual daily activities? Do you need to sleep or rest more than usual?"

Past Health History

A detailed summary of a patient's past health is an important part of the health history. The purpose of the past health history is to compare it with the patient's present respiratory status or uncover risk factors that might predispose him or her to respiratory disorders. Be sure to follow up on any unclear or vague answers. Rewording the question may help the patient find a relevant response.

Family History

The purpose of the family history is to identify any predisposing or causative factors of respiratory origin. If possible, help patients draw a family tree. This helps them remember more relevant information about family members.

Review of Systems

The review of systems (ROS) is used to obtain the current and past health status of each system and to identify health problems that the patient may have failed to mention previously. Changes in the respiratory system have an impact on every other body system. In addition to helping you detect problems that directly affect the respiratory system; the ROS identifies changes in other systems that result from changes in the respiratory system. The ROS allows you to catch anything that you might have missed so far, and it gives meaning to the symptom by relating it to the affected system.

Psychosocial Profile

The psychosocial profile reveals lifestyle patterns that may affect the respiratory system and place the patient at risk for respiratory disorders. The patient's lifestyle may be affected by respiratory disease, especially when it is chronic.

New Words

dyspnea [disp'ni:ə] *n.*　　　　　　　　　　　　　呼吸困难

confusion [kən'fjuːʒn] *n.*	混淆；混乱；困惑
patent ['pætnt] *adj.*	开放的；未闭的；不阻塞的
pleura ['plʊrə] *n.*	喉；喉头
larynx ['lærɪŋks] *n.*	胸膜；肋膜
acoustic [ə'kuːstɪk] *adj.*	听觉的
pharynx ['færɪŋks] *n.*	咽
diaphragm ['daɪəfræm] *n.*	横膈膜
cardiopulmonary [ˌkɑːdɪəʊ'pʌlmənərɪ] *adj.*	心肺的
neuromuscular [ˌnjʊərəʊ'mʌskjʊlər] *adj.*	神经肌肉的
fatigue [fə'tiːg] *n.*	疲劳；疲乏
swelling ['swelɪŋ] *n.*	肿胀；膨胀；增大
hypoxia [haɪ'pɒksɪə] *n.*	低氧；组织缺氧；氧不足
predispose ['priːdɪ'spəʊz] *vt.*	预先处置；使……偏向于

TEXT B　Physical Assessment

The basic human senses are vision, hearing, touch, and smell. These senses may be augmented by special tools (eg. stethoscope, ophthalmoscope, reflex hammer) used in the four fundamental techniques of the physical examination. They are inspection, palpation, percussion, and auscultation. Usually, the four techniques are performed in this order, with the exception of the abdominal assessment. In this case, auscultation precedes palpation and percussion so as not to alter the bowel sounds.

Inspection

The first fundamental technique is inspection or observation. With inspection, a nurse must be sure there is adequate lighting, and must sufficiently expose the area being assessed. Also, the nurse needs to inspect the patient systematically (working from head to toe). Inspection may be direct or indirect. Direct inspection involves directly looking at the patient. Indirect inspection involves using equipment to enhance visualization. For example, specula, such as the nasal speculum and vaginal speculum, open and illuminate, allowing for better visualization.

After systematical inspection, the findings are documented in the patient's chart or health record. Among general observations that should be noted in the initial examination of the patient are posture and stature, body movements, nutritional status, speech pattern, and vital signs.

Palpation

Palpation is a vital part of the physical examination. It usually follows inspection, but both techniques are often performed simultaneously. During palpation, nurses use the sense of touch to collect data. Many structures of the body, although not visible, can be assessed through the techniques of light and deep palpation. Examples include the superficial blood vessels, lymph nodes, thyroid gland, and organs of the abdomen. Furthermore, sounds generated within the body, if within specified frequency ranges, also may be detected through touch. For example, certain murmurs generated in the heart or within blood vessels (thrills) may be detected. Thrills cause a sensation to the hand much like the purring of a cat.

There are two types of palpation, light and deep. Light palpation, which is applying very gentle pressure with the tips and pads of fingers to a body area and then gently moving them over the area, pressing about 1/2 inch, is best for assessing surface characteristics. On the other hand, deep palpation is used to assess organ size, detect masses, and further assess areas of tenderness. And it applies greater pressure with finger tips or pads over an area to a depth greater than 1/2 inch. Moreover, for assessing a partially free-floating object, ballottement is required. The nurse should observe the patient's face during palpation to see if palpation of any area causes discomfort as this may be important in diagnosing a patient's problem. Furthermore, if the nurse knows in advance that the patient is experiencing pain, the painful area should be palpated last.

Percussion

The technique of percussion translates the application of a tap into sound. It is used to assess density of underlying structures, areas of tenderness, and deep tendon reflexes (DTRs). It entails striking a body surface with quick, light blows and eliciting vibrations and sounds.

The sound depends on the density of the underlying tissue and whether it is solid tissue or filled with air or fluid. Two factors influence the sound produced during percussion—the thickness of the surface being perused and the technique. These sounds, listed in a sequence that proceeds from the least to the most dense, are tympany, hyperresonance, resonance, dullness, and flatness. Tympany is the drum-like sound produced by perusing the air-filled stomach. Hyperresonance is audible when one percusses over hyper-inflated lung tissue in a person with emphysema. Resonance is the sound elicited over air-filled lungs. Percussion of the liver produces a dull sound, whereas percussion of bone produces a flat sound. Proper percussion allows the nurse to "outline" the size and shape of the underlying structure.

Auscultation

Auscultation involves using the nurse's hearing to collect data. The nurse listens to sounds produced by the body, such as heart sounds, lung sounds, bowel sounds, and vascular sounds.

Auscultation can be both direct and indirect. Direct auscultation is listening for sounds without a stethoscope, but only a few sounds can be heard in this way. Two examples are respiratory congestion in a patient who requires suctioning and the loud audible murmur of mitral valve replacement.

For most of the sounds produced by the body, nurses need to perform indirect auscultation with a stethoscope. Two end-pieces are available for the stethoscope: the bell and the diaphragm. The bell is used to assess very-low-frequency sounds such as diastolic heart murmurs. The entire surface of the bell's disk is placed lightly on the skin surface to avoid flattening the skin and reducing audible vibratory sensations. The diaphragm, the larger disk, is used to assess high-frequency sounds such as heart and lung sounds and is held in firm contact with the skin surface. Touching the tubing or rubbing other surfaces (hair, clothing) during auscultation needs to be avoided to minimize extraneous noises.

Expertise comes with practice and practice makes perfect. The four physical assessment techniques require nurses to do a lot of practice. Only after having mastered these fundamental techniques, can nurses perform the best possible assessment on their patients.

New Words

stethoscope ['steθəskəʊp] *n.*		听诊器
ophthalmoscope [ɒp'θælməskəʊp] *n.*		检眼镜
inspection [ɪn'spekʃn] *n.*		视诊

palpation [pæl'peɪʃn] *n.*	触诊
percussion [pə'kʌʃn] *n.*	叩诊
auscultation [ˌɔːskəl'teɪʃn] *n.*	听诊
specula ['spekjʊlə] *n.*	反射镜；诊视镜
nasal ['neɪzl] *adj.*	鼻的
vaginal [və'dʒaɪnl] *adj.*	阴道的
illuminate [ɪ'luːmɪneɪt] *v.*	阐明；照亮
lymph [lɪmf] *n.*	淋巴；淋巴液
thyroid ['θaɪrɔɪd] *n.*	甲状腺
murmur ['mɜ˞mər] *n.*	低语；杂音
thrill [θrɪl] *v.*	颤抖；震颤
ballottement [bæ'lɒtmənt] *n.*	冲击触诊法
elicit [ɪ'lɪsɪt] *v.*	抽出；引出
tympany ['tɪmpənɪ] *n.*	鼓音
hyperresonance [ˌhaɪpə'rezənəns] *n.*	过清音
resonance ['rezənəns] *n.*	清音
Dullness ['dʌlnəs] *n.*	浊音
emphysema [ˌemfɪ'siːmə] *n.*	肺气肿
audible ['ɔːdəbl] *adj.*	听得见的
mitral ['maɪtrəl] *adj.*	二尖瓣的
vibratory ['vaɪbrəˌtərɪ] *adj.*	振动的
extraneous [ɪk'streɪnɪəs] *adj.*	外部的

FOLLOW–UP ACTIVITIES

Translation

A.Translate the following sentences into Chinese.

1. The history of the current health concern or illness is the most important factor in helping the health care providers arrive at a diagnosis or determine the patient's needs.

_____

_____

2. Dyspnea may be normal with anxiety, but it may also signal underlying cardiopulmonary or neuromuscular problems or allergic reactions.

_____

_____

3. Light palpation, which is applying very gentle pressure with the tips and pads of fingers to a body area and then gently moving them over the area, pressing about 1/2 inch, is best for assessing surface characteristics.

_____

_____

4. If you notice signs of respiratory distress, such as shortness of breath (SOB), confusion, or anxiety, postpone the detailed history and focus on the acute problem.

_____

_____

5. The review of systems (ROS) is used to obtain the current and past health status of each system and to identify health problems that the patient may have failed to mention previously.

_____

_____

B. Translate the following paragraphs into English.

1. 由于年幼儿童的气道发育不全，免疫功能不健全，因此他们对呼吸道感染疾病更易感。但是，随着年龄的增长，他们的用力呼气量会有所降低，因此呼吸道疾病的发生频次也会降低。

_____

_____

2. 缺氧、呼吸时能量消耗增加，以及相应的心脏损害，会伴有长期的肺部疾病，产生疲乏。

_____

_____

3. 在总体观察时，对患者的初步检查应记录患者的姿势和身高、肢体活动、营养状况、语言模式以及生命体征。

_____

_____

4. 在触诊的过程中，护士必须观察患者的面部，以便发现触诊哪些部位会出现不适，因为这对于诊断患者的疾病可能会很重要。

_____

_____

Unit Four
Clinical Observation

扫一扫，查阅本章数字资源，含PPT、音视频、图片等

After studying this unit, you are required to:

● master basic nursing knowledge of clinical observation, such as the content, the abnormal signs and symptoms of vital signs as well as affected factors and other related terms

● be able to check vital signs for a foreign patient in English, and to judge the meaning of the vital signs

● understand the definition, epidemiology, clinical presentation, investigation and treatment of angina

Part Ⅰ Listening & Speaking

Task 1 Listening

1. Watch the video and discuss the following questions in pairs.

1) What vital signs does nurse 2 (Heather) check for the patient?

2) Why does the doctor confirm that the patient has pneumonia?

3) According to the patient's presentation, what side effects does penicillin have?

4) What medicine has the patient taken?

2. The doctor is examining Miss Jones. Listen to the conversation and answer the following questions.

1) Is Dr. Lynn checking the patient's vital signs?

2) Why does the doctor tell Miss Jones she is in good hands?

3) Has Miss Jones had any nausea or vomiting?

4) How long does Miss Jones wait for the test result?

5) Does nurse 2 (Heather) expose the patient's chest in front of all the people present?

3. In groups, prepare for nurse-patient and doctor-patient interviews. Student A (a doctor), Student B (a nurse) and Student C (a patient) look at the following form, and try to complete the interviews using the information in the form.

Patient's details	Body temperature	
	Chest pain	
	Family doctor	

Doctor's details	Name	
	Department	
	Intravenous drug	
	Effect of Tylenol	

4. In pairs, discuss how you might check vital signs for the following patients.

1) An elderly patient with hypertension

2) A young patient with symptoms of chest pain

Task 2 Dialogue

In pairs, practice the following dialogue and remember the useful words and expressions.

TAKING VITAL SIGNS

(N: Nurse　　　P: Patient)

N: Hello, Mr. Chen. I am going to check your vital signs.

P: Ok. What are vital signs?

N: Your temperature, heart rate, respiratory rate and blood pressure. Please open your mouth. Thanks.

P: How is my temperature?

N: Thirty seven degrees. It's normal. I'll also check your pulse rate.

P: How is my pulse rate?

N: 70 times per minute. It's normal. Let me take your blood pressure now.

P: What's my blood pressure?

N: 140 mmHg over 90 mmHg.

P: Is that normal?

N: It's higher than normal. Now I'll check your respiratory rate. Please unbutton your shirt, and lie down on your back. Please breathe normally.

P: How is it?

N: It is 18 times per minute; it's normal. Now let me listen to your heart and lungs. Take a deep breath in… and out… now hold your breath, again. Ok, you can breathe again normally now. Thank you!

P: How's everything?

N: There are cardiac murmurs. Don't worry too much. Cardiac murmurs do not necessarily mean that you have a heart disease. It might be just a temporary physiological condition.

P: I was told that I had cardiac murmurs during the physical examination.

N: I think it is a physiological condition. You can take the Doppler echocardiograph for a more accurate diagnosis. Your vital signs, except your blood pressure and cardiac murmurs, are all normal. Okay, so much for your vital signs.

Part Ⅱ　Reading

Reading Guidance

Is it necessary for a nurse to learn to do clinical observation? What are vital signs? Is it

important for a nurse to check a patient's vital signs? Monitoring vital signs is an important nursing assessment. Yet, nurses seem to do it as a routine and they often overlook its significance in recognizing a patient's disease. Clinical observation, including vital signs, plays a critical role in the assessment of the patient's condition, especially in emergency departments. It is especially important for a nurse to observe symptoms and check the vital signs of patients with coronary artery disease, especially the changes of heart rate at any time.

Before Class
Please think about these questions carefully and discuss with your classmates.

● How important is clinical observation for nurses?

● How do you evaluate nurses' ability of clinical observation in your country?

● How can nurses improve their clinical observation ability?

TEXT A   Vital Signs

Vital signs include body temperature, pulse rate and rhythm, respiration, and blood pressure. Any changes in vital signs may indicate changes in health. Vital signs should be measured when the patient is in a resting state. Any abnormal findings should be measured again in order to verify the findings.

Frequency of Measuring Vital Signs

Vital signs are measured at least every 4 hours in hospitalized patients who have low or high blood pressures, and/or elevated temperatures, and/or variations in pulse rate or rhythm, and/or respiratory difficulty, and in patients who had a surgery or who are receiving medicines that would affect cardiovascular or respiratory function.

Times to Assess Vital Signs

● On admission to obtain baseline medical data

● When a patient has abnormal symptoms such as fever, chest pain or palpitation, etc.

● Before and after surgery or an invasive procedure

● Before and/or after the administration of a medication that could affect the cardiovascular or respiratory systems, such as before giving digitalis preparation

● Before and after any nursing interventions that could affect the vital signs such as moving a patient who has been on bed rest

Body Temperature

Body temperature is assessed with a thermometer. It reflects the dynamic balance between the heat produced and heat lost from the body. Normal range for body temperature is 36.1°C to 37.8°C. There are a number of factors that can affect the body temperature, such as circadian rhythms, stress, exercise, environmental temperature, age and hormones. The most common sites for measuring body temperature include the oral, axillary, rectal and the tympanic membrane (in ear). Usually, body temperature is lower in the morning than it is in late afternoon and evening. Common abnormal body temperature includes hyperthermia, hyperpyrexia and hypothermia, etc.

● **Hyperthermia** A body temperature above the normal range, also called pyrexia or fever.

● **Hyperpyrexia** A very high fever usually above 41℃ ; if the body temperature reaches 44.0℃ , survival is rare. Death will occur due to damaging effects on the respiratory center.

● **Hypothermia** A condition in which core temperature or internal temperature falls below 35℃. It is below the required temperature for normal metabolism and functions of the human body. A body temperature below 35℃ is a medical emergency and can lead to death if not treated promptly.

Pulse Rate and Rhythm

The pulse is created by contraction of the left ventricle of the heart. Pulse rate is measured by counting the number of heart contractions in one minute. Pulse can be checked at the wrist (radial pulse) or at the neck (carotid pulse). A resting adult heart rate should be between 60 and 100 beats per minute. It can be affected by age, gender, exercise, medication and fever, etc. Athletes may have lower rates. Children will have higher pulse rates. And in normal conditions, heart rhythm should be regular, without any missing or closely spaced beats. The common abnormal pulses include:

● **Tachycardia** An excessively fast heart rate: over 100 beats per minute (BPM) in an adult.

● **Bradycardia** A heart rate less than 60 BPM in an adult.

● **Dysrhythmia** or Arrhythmia A pulse with an irregular rhythm.

Respiratory

● **Respiratory rate**

Respiratory rate is the number of breaths in one minute when the patient is at rest. To do this, count the number of times the chest rises for one full minute while the patient is breathing normally. The normal adult rate is 12 to 18 breaths per minute. Children breathe faster. There are some terms about respiration as follows:

Eupnea Normal in depth and rate.

Bradypnea Abnormally slow respiration.

Tachypnea Abnormally fast respiration.

Apnea The absence of breathing.

● **Breath sounds**

Stridor Harsh sound heard during inspiration with laryngeal obstruction.

Wheeze Continuous, high pitched musical sound occurring on expiration when air moves through a narrowed or partially obstructed airway.

● **Secretions and coughing**

Hemoptysis The presence of blood in the sputum.

Productive cough A cough accompanied by expectorated secretions.

Nonproductive cough A dry, harsh cough without secretions.

Blood Pressure

Blood pressure is the force of the blood against arterial walls. It consists of two aspects, i.e. systolic pressure and diastolic pressure. The former means the maximum blood pressure exerted on the walls of arteries when the left ventricles of the heart push blood through the aortic valve into the arteries during contraction. Diastolic pressure is the pressure when the ventricles relax. The difference between systolic and diastolic pressure is called the pulse pressure. Blood pressure can be affected by age, stress, obesity, gender, race and medications. The average blood pressure is 120 over 80 mmHg. A resting blood pressure of over 90 diastolic is considered mildly elevated; over 100 may require treatment.

- **Hypertension** An abnormal high blood pressure, over 140 mmHg systolic and 90 mmHg diastolic.
- **Hypotension** Blood pressure below normal, between 85-110 mmHg systolic.

New Words

axillary [æk'sɪlərɪ] *adj.*	腋窝的
tympanic [tɪm'pænɪk] *adj.*	鼓膜的
hyperthermia [ˌhaɪpə'θɜ:mɪə] *n.*	过高热，极高热
hyperpyrexia [ˌhaɪpəpaɪ'reksɪə] *n.*	高热，体温过高
hypothermia [ˌhaɪpə'θɜ:mɪə] *n.*	体温过低
tachycardia [ˌtækɪ'kɑ:dɪə] *n.*	心动过速
bradycardia [ˌbrædɪ'kɑ:dɪə] *n.*	心动过缓
arrhythmia [eɪ'rɪðmɪə] *n.*	心律不齐
bradypnea [bræ'dipnɪə] *n.*	呼吸过慢
tachypnea [ˌtækɪp'nɪə] *n.*	呼吸促迫，呼吸急促
stridor ['straɪdə] *n.*	喘鸣
hemoptysis [hɪ'mɒptɪsɪs] *n.*	咳血，咯血
systolic [ˌsɪ'stɒlɪk] *adj.*	心脏收缩（期）的
diastolic [ˌdaɪə'stɒlɪk] *adj.*	心脏舒张（期）的
hypertension [ˌhaɪpə'tenʃn] *n.*	高血压
hypotension [haɪpə(ʊ)'tenʃ(ə)n] *n.*	低血压

TEXT B   Angina

Angina is chest pain or discomfort which arises from areas of cardiac muscle which are underperfused and lack adequate supply of oxygen. Angina may be caused by:

. a fixed stenosis (>50%) of one or more coronary arteries

. coronary artery spasm

. diseases other than IHD, e.g. aortic stenosis

Epidemiology

Mortality of coronary heart disease

According to the most recent data published by the American Heart Association, coronary heart disease (CHD) alone caused approximately one of every six deaths in the USA in 2009. On the basis of data from the National Health and Nutrition Examination Survey 2007–2010, an estimated 15.4 million Americans have CHD, with a prevalence of 6.4% in the US population.

Prevalence of angina

In the United States, an analysis of studies of acute coronary syndrome (ACS) led to an estimate of 16.5 million people with angina (prevalence of 5.3%) . The weighted prevalence of definite angina (Rose) in the Spanish population aged 40 years or older was 2.6% and was higher in women (2.9%) than in men (2.2%), whereas that of confirmed angina was 1.4%, without differences between men (1.5%) and women (1.3%). The prevalence of definite angina (Rose) increased with age (0.7% in patients aged 40 to 49 years and 7.1% in those aged 70 years or older). Both prevalences increased with age, cardiovascular risk factors, and cardiovascular history.

It is estimated that nearly 8 million people in the United States (US) suffer from chronic stable angina. Chronic stable angina (CSA) is usually described as predictable chest pain on exertion or when under mental or emotional stress. Estimates from the National Health and Nutrition Examination Survey 2007–2010 show a prevalence of CSA of 7.8 million people (3.2% of the US population). The annual rates per 1,000 population of new episodes of CSA for non-black men are 28.3 for those aged 65–74 years, 36.3 for those aged 75–84 years, and 33.0 for those aged ≥85 years.

Clinical presentation

Symptoms

Typically it is a central, crushing chest pain, of variable severity. Classically it radiates to the jaw and left arm or into the neck. It is often worse when

- exercising in cold air

- anxious

- hurrying

- angry

It is relieved with rest and sublingual nitroglycerin. In some individuals the pain may be less apparent and the sensation is more of chest tightness and breathlessness (dyspnoea). Anginal pain may come on when lying down at night (decubitus angina, caused by increased venous return in patients with incipient heart failure) or at rest (fixed coronary atheromatous disease or coronary artery spasm).

Signs

You should examine patients carefully and keep in mind the cardiovascular and systemic diseases that can disturb the balance of oxygen supply and demand (e.g. aortic stenosis, anaemia). Look for risk factors such as hypertension. Patients with IHD may have signs of heart failure or peripheral vascular disease, but many will have no abnormal signs at all.

The relationship between frequency of episodes of painless ischemia and BP level in patients with stable effort angina was J-shaped: sensitivity to ischemia was lowered and frequency of painless ischemia increased both at highest and lowest values of BP.

Investigations

The characteristics of the electrocardiogram (ECG)

The resting ECG may show ST segment or T wave changes suggestive of ischemia, or evidence of unsuspected previous myocardial infarction or hypertension, but it is often normal. It is most likely to be abnormal if recorded when the patient is in "pain".

Exercise testing

Exercise can be used to provoke symptomatic or asymptomatic ECG changes that are absent at rest. After recording a baseline ECG, the patient is exercised on a treadmill or bicycle ergometer and the work load serially increased under medical supervision with resuscitation facilities immediately at hand.

The following are criteria for a positive response:

- horizontal or down sloping ST segment depression>2mm

- typical ischaemic symptoms

- dysrhythmias

● a fall in blood pressure.

The result is expressed as a probability of IHD, recognizing that some patients with IHD have negative tests and that minor ST segment changes may develop in patients without IHD. Exercise testing is contraindicated immediately after acute myocardial infarction and in uncontrolled hypertension, severe aortic stenosis and unstable angina.

Coronary angiography

Imaging the coronary arteries after injection of a radiographic contrast medium into them is the "gold standard" investigation to detect atherosclerotic disease of the coronary arteries. Coronary angiography can reliably assess the severity of coronary atherosclerosis and exclude its presence but cannot absolutely exclude ischaemia as the cause of chest pain. Myocardial perfusion scanning may be diagnostic of coronary ischaemia in patients with normal coronary arteries.

Drugs used in the management of angina

Strategies for the treatment of angina can be targeted at either increasing the coronary blood flow or decreasing the work done by the heart. In the latter case oxygen demand is decreased. This can be achieved by reducing the force of cardiac muscle contraction either by reducing preload on the heart or by reducing cardiac contractility. Other changes in workload of the heart can be achieved by reducing heart rate or arterial blood pressure (decreased afterload).

Four major classes of drugs are used:

● organic nitrates, such as glyceryl trinitrate, isosorbide dinitrate and isosorbide mononitrate.

● ß-adrenocepter blockers, such as atenolol, propranolol.

● calcium channel blockers, such as nifedipine, amLodipine, verapamil and diltiazem.

● potassium channel openers, such as nicorandil.

New Words

angina [æn'dʒaɪnə] *n.*	心绞痛
stenosis [stɪ'nəʊsɪs] *n.*	（器官）狭窄
coronary ['kɒrənri] *adj.*	冠状的，（心脏的）冠状动脉的
cardiovascular [ˌkɑːdiəʊ'væskjələ(r)] *adj.*	心血管的
dyspnoea [dɪsp'niː ə] *n.*	呼吸困难
atheromatous [ˌæθə'rɑmətəs] *adj.*	动脉粥样化的
infarction [ɪn'fɑːkʃn] *n.*	梗死；梗死形成
radiographic [ˌreɪdɪəʊ'græfɪk] *adj.*	射线照相术的

FOLLOW–UP ACTIVITIES

Translation

A. Translate the following sentences into Chinese.

1. Vital signs are body temperature, pulse rate and rhythm, respiration, and blood pressure.

2. Body temperature is assessed with a thermometer. It reflects the dynamic balance between the heat produced and heat lost from the body.

_____

_____

3. There are a number of factors that can affect the body temperature, such as circadian rhythms, stress, exercise, environmental temperature, age and hormones, etc.

_____

_____

4. There are some terms about respiration as follows: Eupnea, Bradypnea, Tachypnea, Apnea, breath sounds, secretions and coughing.

_____

_____

B. Translate the following paragraphs into English.

1. 脉率通常在腕部桡动脉处检查，并以每分钟跳动次数记录，或用听诊器直接听诊心脏而获取。脉率随着年龄发生变化。成年人通常 60 ～ 100 次 / 分，而新生儿每分钟则可达 130 ～ 150 次。

_____

_____

2. 生命体征是检测各种生理状况以评估人体基础功能的指标。异常生命体征表明健康状况出现变化。生命体征常随着年龄而发生改变。

_____

_____

3. 血压是指血液作用于动脉壁的压力。它包括两个方面，即收缩压和舒张压。前者是在心脏收缩期，左心室的血液经过主动脉瓣泵入主动脉时，血液对血管壁产生的最大侧压力。

_____

_____

4. 呼吸频率是患者休息时每分钟呼吸的次数，可以通过一分钟胸部起伏的总次数来计数。正常成人呼吸频率是每分钟 12 至 18 次。

_____

_____

扫一扫，查阅本
章数字资源，含
PPT、音视频、
图片等

After studying this unit, you are required to:

- **explain the definition of pain**
- **master the basic knowledge of cancer pain**
- **be able to assess pain for a foreign patient in English**

Part I Listening & Speaking

Task 1 Video Watching

1. Watch the video on assessment of symptoms and pain; and then discuss the following questions in pairs.

1) What does "PQRST" stand for in assessing symptoms?

2) How can we know that a patient's shortness-of-breath is getting worse?

3) What does "WILDA" stand for in assessing pain?

4) How can we assess the intensity of pain?

5) What questions can we ask to assess the duration of pain?

2. Heather, the ward nurse, is assessing pain for Mrs. Smith. Listen to the conversation and answer the following questions.

1) Where is the pain?

2) What does the pain feel like?

3) On a scale of 1 to 10, how does the patient rate the pain?

4) What strategy will the nurse use to relieve the pain?

5) What probably causes the pain on the back of the patient's leg?

3. In pairs, prepare to do a pain assessment. Student A, the nurse, please look at the Pain Assessment Form and think about the questions you will ask to complete it. Student B, the patient who suffers from appendicitis, please imagine the pain you might feel and be ready to answer the nurse's questions in detail.

PAIN ASSESSMENT FORM

Location		
Onset		
Type		
Radiation		
Associated symptoms		
Duration		
Intensity		
Offset		

4. In pairs, discuss the following questions.

1) Are you good at dealing with pain?

2) Do you have any special ways to deal with pain?

3) Do you have any experience of looking after someone in pain?

Task 2 Dialogue

In pairs, practice the following dialogue and remember the useful words and expressions.

PAIN ASSESSMENT

(N: Nurse   P: Patient)

P: It hurts. Could you please help me, nurse?

N: Sure. But before I call a doctor, I'd like to ask you a few questions. Tell me where your pain is, please?

P: In my right lower tummy, here.

N: OK. Please tell me how your pain feels? Is it sharp, dull, or aching?

P: It is a sharp pain.

N: I see. Now I want to know whether your pain is mild, moderate or severe. Let's say, on a scale of 0 to 10, "0" is when you feel no pain and "10" is when you feel the worst possible pain. How would you rate the degree of your pain?

P: Eight, I guess.

N: That is quite a lot of pain. Just a few more questions, when did the pain start?

P: Last night, around 10 o'clock.

N: Was it sudden or gradual?

P: It was sudden. I was watching a television program at that time.

N: What makes the pain worse?

P: When I move or sit in a chair, it gets even worse.

N: OK. What have you tried to relieve the pain? Has anything worked?

P: I took a pain-killer, an aspirin before I came here. I felt a little bit better after that and I fell asleep for 2 or 3 hours. But the pain started again early this morning.

N: I see. Do you have any other symptoms associated with the pain?

P: I felt nausea and vomited a few times around 5: 30 this morning.

N: How does the pain affect your sleep and appetite?

P: I didn't sleep well last night and I didn't eat anything for breakfast this morning.

N: I see. I will arrange for a doctor to see you very soon.

P: Thank you.

Part II Reading

Reading Guidance

Pain is an unpleasant emotional experience as well as an uncomfortable physical sensation. It happens when parts of the body are damaged. This damage irritates nerve endings, which then send a warning signal to the brain. The brain responds by making us feel pain or discomfort. For people with cancer, pain is a common experience. What causes pain for cancer patients? How does it affect cancer patients' quality of life? What can be done to have cancer pain treated? Why haven't some cancer patients received adequate treatment for cancer pain? Nurses spend more time with patients than any other members of the healthcare team. They play a critical, active, and very important role in controlling cancer patients' pain and alleviating their suffering.

Before Class

Please think carefully about these questions and discuss with your classmates.

- **What causes pain for cancer patients?**

- **What aspects of cancer patients' life will be affected by cancer pain?**

- **How can nurses manage pain for cancer patients?**

- **Why is cancer pain often undertreated?**

TEXT A   Cancer Pain

To many people, the word "cancer" means pain and death. Unfortunately, there is much to support this view. One study found that 30% of patients experience pain at the time of diagnosis, 30%–50% experience pain while undergoing treatment, and 70%–90% experience pain as cancer advances. To achieve the goal of providing adequate pain relief for patients with cancer, healthcare providers seek to understand the causes and types of cancer pain, its impact on patients' life, and treatment of cancer pain.

Causes of Cancer Pain

Most cancer pain is caused by the tumor itself, be it the primary tumor (where the tumor started) or the metastatic tumor (where the tumor has spread). Cancer can cause pain by growing into or destroying tissues near the cancer, and by pressing on bones, nerves or other organs in a patient's body. Sometimes pain is related to cancer treatment. Surgery causes pain, as tissues are cut or damaged. Radiotherapy can damage the skin in the area being treated, causing a burning sensation or painful scars. Chemotherapy can damage the soft tissues in the mouth, causing soreness. In addition, other factors such as fear, anxiety, depression and a lack of sleep can also make patients' pain worse.

Types of Cancer Pain

Cancer pain can be acute or chronic. Acute pain starts suddenly, is usually sharp in nature, and of relatively short duration. It is due to damage caused by an injury and ends when the source is removed. For example, having an operation can cause acute pain. The pain disappears when the wound heals. In the meantime, painkillers will usually keep it under control.

Chronic pain on the other hand, has a less distinct onset, a prolonged and fluctuating course. It is usually described as burning or aching in nature and lasts for a long period of time. Chronic pain is caused by changes to nerves. Nerve changes may occur due to cancer pressing on nerves or due to chemicals produced by a tumor. It can also be caused by nerve changes due to cancer treatment. The pain continues long after the injury or treatment is over and can range from mild to severe. It can be there all the time and requires careful, ongoing attention to be appropriately treated.

Quality of Life Issues

Pain can greatly affect cancer patients' quality of life. The list of damage that pain does to quality of life includes:

- Sleep is disturbed.
- Ability to work is impaired.
- Exhaustion can become a constant companion.
- Sadness, depression and worry are commonly felt emotions.
- Appetite diminishes.
- Simple pleasures such as enjoying one's family are impaired or given up.
- Trips and vacations are uncomfortable or impossible.
- Reluctance to move or exercise is experienced.
- Feelings of isolation from the world increase.

Treatment of Cancer Pain

There are many different ways to treat cancer pain. One way is to remove the source of the pain, for example, through surgery, chemotherapy, radiation or some other forms of treatment. If that can't be done, pain medications can usually control the pain. These medications include:

- Over-the-counter (OTC) and prescription-strength pain relievers, such as aspirin, acetaminophen and ibuprofen.
- Weak opioid (derived from opium) medications, such as codeine.
- Strong opioid medications, such as morphine, oxycodone, hydromorphone, fentanyl, methadone or oxymorphone.

These drugs can often be taken orally, so they're easy to use. Medications may come in tablet form, or they may be made to dissolve quickly in your mouth. However, if you're unable to take medications orally, they may also be taken intravenously, rectally or through the skin using a patch.

Specialized treatment, such as nerve blocks, may also be used. Nerve blocks are a local anesthetic that is injected around or into a nerve, which prevents pain messages traveling along that nerve pathway from reaching the brain.

Other therapies such as acupuncture, acupressure, massage, physical therapy, relaxation, meditation and humor may help.

Reasons for Under-treatment of Cancer Pain

Remember, cancer pain can be managed. With today's knowledge of cancer pain and the availability of pain-relieving therapies, no one should have to suffer from unrelieved pain. Although cancer pain can be relieved, surveys have shown that pain is often undertreated. Many factors may contribute to that, some of which include:

● **Physicians may not be adequately educated about pain control.** Some doctors don't know enough about proper pain treatment. Others may be concerned about prescribing pain medications because these drugs can be abused. However, people in pain are very unlikely to abuse pain medications.

● **Reluctance of doctors to ask about pain or offer treatments.** Some doctors and other health care professionals may focus more on the control of disease than on the control of pain; they may not specifically ask about pain, which should be a normal part of every visit.

● **Reluctance of patients to report their pain.** A third factor might be a person's own reluctance. Some people might not want to "bother" their doctors with the information, or they may fear that the pain means that their cancer is getting worse. They might feel that because they have cancer, they're supposed to have pain and bear it. That simply isn't true.

● **Fear of addiction.** Another factor might be a person's fear of becoming addicted to pain medications. This is something that we know doesn't typically happen if patients take pain medications for pain in an appropriate fashion.

● **Fear of side effects.** Some people fear the side effects of pain medications. Many are afraid of being sleepy, being unable to communicate with family and friends, acting strangely, or being seen as dependent on medications. People are also sometimes afraid that taking morphine may shorten their life. There is no evidence of any of these happenings if the medication is dosed appropriately.

New Words

metastatic [ˌmetə'stætɪk] *adj.*	转移性的；转移的
radiotherapy [reɪdiəʊ'θerəpi] *n.*	放射治疗
chemotherapy [kiːməʊ'θerəpi] *n.*	化学疗法；化学药物治疗
acute [ə'kjuːt] *adj.*	急性的；敏锐的；激烈的
chronic ['krɒnɪk] *adj.*	慢性的；长期的；习惯性的
painkiller ['peɪnkɪlə(r)] *n.*	止痛药
exhaustion [ɪg'zɔːstʃən] *n.*	枯竭；耗尽；精疲力竭
over-the-counter [əʊvəðə 'kaʊntə(r)] *adj.*	［医］非处方药的
prescription [prɪ'skrɪpʃn] *n.*	处方
opioid ['əʊpɪɔɪd] *n.*	鸦片样物质；类鸦片
intravenously [ɪntrə'viːnəsli] *adv.*	静脉注射地；通过静脉
rectally ['rɛktli] *adv.*	直肠给药地
anesthetic [ænɪsθetɪk] *n.*	麻醉剂；麻药
acupuncture ['ækjupʌŋktʃə(r)] *n.*	针刺疗法

Please think carefully about these questions and discuss with your classmates.

- **What is the definition of pain?**

- **What are the five key elements of pain assessment?**

- **How do you assess a patient's pain intensity by using 0-10 numeric scale?**

TEXT B   How to Assess Pain

According to the International Association for the Study of Pain, pain is an unpleasant sensory and emotional experience arising from actual or potential tissue damage. Clinically, pain is a subjective experience and the only person who truly knows what the pain is like is the one who is having it.

Pain is a red flag. It tells us there is a problem somewhere in the body that is crying out for attention. Careful, comprehensive pain assessment is critical to optimal pain management. Many health care facilities are making pain assessment the fifth vital sign.

Pain assessment should be ongoing, individualized, and documented so that all those involved in the patient's care can understand the pain problem. Using the WILDA approach ensures that the five key elements of pain assessment are incorporated into the process.

Pain assessment usually begins with an open-ended question: "Tell me about your pain." This allows the patient to tell his or her story, including the aspects of the pain experience that are most problematic. The nurse must listen closely to these first words. Patients in pain want to tell their stories, and nurses need to take time to listen.

Words

A patient's simple statement, like "I have pain", is not descriptive enough. Asking patients to describe their pain using words will guide nurses to the appropriate interventions for specific pain types. The following questions should be asked of patients:

- What does your pain feel like?

- Because various pain types are described using different words, what words would you use to describe the pain you are having?

Intensity

The ability to quantify the intensity of pain is essential when caring for patients with pain. Dalton and McNaull advocate a universal adoption of a 0 to 10 scale for clinical assessment of pain intensity in adult patients. Using a pain scale with 0 being no pain and 10 being the worst possible pain, a numerical value can be assigned to the patient's perceived intensity of pain. Another way to assess the intensity of pain is the Visual Analog Scale (VAS). It is a 100-millimeter line with "no pain" on one end and "pain as bad as it can be" at the other end. Patients are expected to mark on the line the amount of pain they are experiencing. An additional way to evaluate the intensity of pain is to determine the extent of pain awareness and degrees of interference with functioning. For example, 0=no pain, 2=awareness of pain only when paying attention to it, 4=can ignore pain and do things, 6=can't ignore pain, interferes with functioning, 8=impairs ability to function or concentrate, and 10=intense incapacitating pain. Asking patients to rate their present pain, their pain at the best and worst in the previous 24 hours and the effect of any medications or interventions will enable nurses to see if the pain is worsening or improving. Also, asking about the pain level acceptable to the patient will help nurses understand the patient's expectation of therapy.

Location

Patients can have two or more sources of pain and some pain may radiate to other parts of the body. Thus, it is essential to ask patients, "Where is your pain?" or "Do you have pain in more than one area?" The pain that the patient may be referring to may be different than the one the nurse is talking about. Having the patient point to the painful area can be more specific and help to identify location.

Duration

Pain may be constant or intermittent. Asking the patient, "How long does the pain last?" and/or "Is the pain always there, or does it just come and go?", "How much time do you have between periods of pain?"

Aggravating/Alleviating Factors

The patient should be asked to describe the factors that aggravate or alleviate the pain as this will help in planning interventions. A typical question might be, "What makes the pain better or worse?" Analgesics and non-pharmacologic approaches such as massage, relaxation, music, heat or cold, and nerve blocks may relieve the pain. Other factors such as movement and depression may intensify the pain.

Pain assessment should also include the presence of contributing symptoms or side effects associated with pain and its treatment. These include nausea, vomiting, constipation, sleepiness, confusion, urinary retention, and weakness. Some patients may tolerate these symptoms without aggressive treatment; others may choose to stop taking pain medications because of side effect intolerance.

Inquiring about the presence or absence of changes in appetite, activity, relationships, sexual functioning, irritability, sleep, anxiety, anger, and ability to concentrate will help the nurse to understand the pain experience in each individual. Additionally, the nurses should discern how pain is perceived by the patient and his or her family or significant others and what works and doesn't work to help relieve the pain.

New Words

optimal ['ɒptɪməl] *adj.*	最佳的；最理想的
intervention [ˌɪntə'venʃn] *n.*	干预，介入
quantify ['kwɒntɪfaɪ] *vt.*	量化；为……定量；确定数量
numerical [njuː'merɪkl] *adj.*	数值的；数字的；用数字表示的
interference [ɪntə'fɪərəns] *n.*	干扰；干涉
incapacitate [ˌɪnkə'pæsɪteɪt] *vt.*	使无能力；使不能
radiate ['reɪdieɪt] *vi.*	辐射；从中心向各方伸展
intermittent [ˌɪntə'mɪtənt] *adj.*	间歇的；断断续续的；间歇性
aggravate ['æɡrəveɪt] *vt.*	加重；使恶化；激怒
constipation [ˌkɒnstɪ'peɪʃn] *n.*	便秘
irritability [ɪrɪtə'bɪləti] *n.*	过敏性；易怒；兴奋性

FOLLOW–UP ACTIVITIES

Translation

A. Translate the following sentences into Chinese.

1. Cancer can cause pain by growing into or destroying tissue near the cancer, and by pressing on bones, nerves or other organs in a patient's body.

_____

_____

2. Nerve blocks are a local anesthetic that is injected into or around a nerve, which prevents pain messages traveling along that nerve pathway from reaching the brain.

_____

_____

3. With today's knowledge of cancer pain and the availability of pain-relieving therapies, no one should have to suffer from unrelieved pain.

_____

_____

4. Some doctors and other health care professionals may focus more on the control of disease than on the control of pain; they may not specifically ask about pain, which should be a normal part of every visit.

_____

_____

B. Translate the following paragraphs into English.

1. 标准疼痛评估量表适用于急性疼痛，但对于慢性疼痛患者来说，很难使用数字量表。护士评估患者疼痛是否改善的更佳方法是，每天询问慢性疼痛患者感受到的疼痛程度。对于这些患者，疼痛管理是否成功的衡量标准不是疼痛程度是否减轻，而是患者的功能是否增加。

_____

_____

2. 对患者疼痛的综合评估包括但不局限于以下方面：疼痛的部位、程度及持续时间；加重和减轻疼痛的因素；疼痛对患者日常生活、睡眠模式、心理方面的影响；目前疼痛管理策略的效果。

_____

_____

Medication Administration

扫一扫，查阅本
章数字资源，含
PPT、音视频、
图片等

After studying this unit, you are required to:

● **master the basic knowledge of medication administration**

● **be able to communicate with a foreign patient in English when administering medication**

Part Ⅰ Listening & Speaking

Task 1 Video Watching

1. Watch the video and discuss the following questions in pairs.

1) What are the "seven rights"?

2) What does the nurse do before she offers the treatment to the patient?

3) What does the nurse do when she is administering medication to the patient?

2. Listen to the conversation and answer the following questions.

1) What does the patient say to the nurse before receiving the IV treatment?

2) Does the patient ask for any help after the treatment?

Task 2 Dialogue

In Pairs, practice the following dialogue and remember the useful words and expressions.

ADMINISTERING DIGOXIN TO A HEART FAILURE PATIENT

(N: nurse   P: Patient)

N: Good morning, Mr. Jobs. How do you feel today?

P: Good morning, Cindy. I feel much better.

N: Did you sleep well last night?

P: Much better! I have had trouble sleeping for a while but last night I slept for about 6 hours.

N: Sounds great! It's time for you to take digoxin now. But before I give you the drug, would you please give me your hand, I need to look at your identification bracelet to verify your name and your date of birth (DOB). Your name is…

P: Thomas Jobs.

N: And your DOB is?

P: November 30, 1958.

N: Let me check your pulse. Your pulse is 82 beats per minute, quite normal. So, I am going to give you the medication.

P: Okay. But before you give me the drug, can you repeat the drug name for me?

N: Sure, digoxin, it is also called lanoxin. This is the commonly used digitalis glycoside, and it comes from the plant "fox glove." The drug is used to increase the force of heart contraction.

P: Thanks.

N: Well, which do you prefer, sitting at the bedside or in a chair?

P: Sitting in a chair.

N: Ok, let me assist you. Your doctor has ordered the daily digoxin 0.125mg for you. So I am going to give you a half pill. Here you are. Take a full glass of water to swallow it.

P: Thanks. You are so nice.

N: My pleasure! The call bell is right here, please call me if you need anything. Anyway, I will check back with you in a few minutes.

P: Thank you Cindy. See you.

Part II Reading

Reading Guidance

It is very important for a nurse to grasp the basic principles of administering medication. The essential elements are the three checks and the seven rights which are commonly applied in clinics. What are the three checks and the seven rights? How do nurses apply them in clinics? What is the nursing process involved in medication administration? What are medication errors? How many types of medication errors are there? How can nurses avoid medication errors? You will find the answers in this text.

Before Class

Please think about these questions carefully and discuss with your classmates.

● **What does a nurse do before administering heart failure medication?**

● **Why is it important for a patient to take the heart failure medication at the right time and in the appropriate way?**

● **How can nurses administer medication correctly?**

TEXT A   Heart Failure Medicines

Heart failure is a kind of cardiovascular disease. Most people who have heart failure need to take medicines. Some of these medicines are used to treat patients' symptoms and others may help to prevent their heart failure from becoming worse and let them live longer as well.

As a heart failure patient, you will need to take most of your heart failure medicines every day. Some medicines are taken once a day. Others need to be taken 2 or more times daily. It is very important that you take your medicines at the right time and in the way your doctor has told you.

Never stop taking your heart medicines without talking to your doctor first. This is also true for other medicines you take, such as drugs for diabetes, high blood pressure, and other serious conditions. Nurses play a very important role in administering medication for the patients.

Your doctor may also tell you to take certain medicines. Do not change your medicines or doses without talking to your doctor. Sometimes doctors also need to adjust the medication based on your symptoms. In this regard nurses should keep contact with the patients from time to time.

Always tell your doctor before you take any new medicines. This includes over-the-counter medicines such as ibuprofen (Advil, Motrin) and naproxen (Aleve, Naprosyn), as well as drugs such as sildenafil (Viagra), vardenafil (Levitra), and tadalafil (Cialis).

Also tell your doctor before you take any type of herb or supplement. The more information you tell the doctor the safter you are. After the doctor's comprehensive analysis, you will get the right medication for your diseases.

ACE Inhibitors and ARBs

ACE inhibitors (angiotensin converting enzyme inhibitors) and ARBs (angiotensin II receptor blockers) work by opening blood vessels and lowering blood pressure. These medicines can:

- Reduce the work your heart has to do.
- Help your heart muscle pump better.
- Keep your heart failure from getting worse.
- Prevent or reduce harmful changes to your heart muscle.

Common side effects of these drugs include:

- Dry cough
- Lightheadedness
- Fatigue
- Upset stomach
- Edema
- Headache
- Diarrhea

When you take these medicines, your doctor will order blood tests to check how well your kidneys are working and to measure your potassium levels.

Beta Blockers

Beta blockers slow your heart rate and decrease the strength with which your heart muscle contracts in the short term. Long term beta blockers help keep your heart failure from becoming worse. They may also help strengthen your heart. Common beta blockers used for heart failure include carvedilol (Coreg), bisoprolol (Zebeta), and metoprolol (Toprol). Do not abruptly stop taking these drugs. This can increase the risk of angina and even a heart attack. Other side effects include lightheadedness, depression, fatigue, and memory loss.

Water Pills or Diuretics

Diuretics help your body get rid of extra fluid. Some types of diuretics may also help in other ways. These drugs are often called "water pills". There are many brands of diuretics. Some are taken once a day. Others are taken twice a day. The most common types are:

- Thiazides. Chlorothiazide (Diuril), chlorthalidone (Hygroton), indapamide (Lozol), hydrochlorothiazide (Esidrix, HydroDiuril), and metolazone (Mykrox, Zaroxolyn).

● Loop diuretics. Bumentanide (Bumex), furosemide (Lasix), and torasemide (Demadex).

● Potassium-sparing agents. Amiloride (Midamor), spironolactone (Aldactone), and　　triamterene (Dyrenium).

When you take these medicines, you will need regular blood tests to check how well your kidneys are working and measure your potassium levels.

Other Drugs for Heart Failure

Many people with heart disease take either aspirin or clopidogrel (Plavix). These drugs help to prevent blood clots from forming in your arteries. This can lower your risk of stroke or heart attack. Coumadin (Warfarin) is recommended for patients with heart failure who have a higher risk for blood clots. You will need to have extra blood tests to make sure your dose is correct. You may also need to make changes to your diet.

Drugs used less commonly for heart failure include:

● Digoxin to help increase the heart's pumping strength and slow the heart rate.

● Hydralazine and nitrates to open up arteries and help the heart muscle pump better.

These drugs are mainly used by patients who are unable to tolerate ACE inhibitors and angiotensin receptor blockers.

● Calcium channel blockers to control blood pressure or angina (chest pain) from coronary artery disease (CAD).

Statins and other cholesterol-lowering drugs are used when needed. Antiarrhythmic medicines are sometimes used by heart failure patients who have abnormal heart rhythms, one of which is amiodarone.

No matter what type of heart failure medicine, before you take it, you should always talk to your doctor and nurse about your medication-taking history, your detailed symptoms, medication side effects, and so on.

New Words

diabetes [ˌdaɪə'biːtiːz] *n.*	糖尿病；多尿症
ibuprofen [ˌaɪbjuː'prəʊfen] *n.*	［医］布洛芬，异丁苯丙酸（抗炎镇痛药）
naproxen [nə'prɒksɛn] *n.*	萘普生；甲氧萘丙酸
convert [kən'vɜːt] *vt.*	（使）转变；使皈依；兑换，换算
enzyme ['enzaɪm] *n.*	［生化］酶
inhibitor [ɪn'hɪbɪtə(r)] *n.*	抑制剂，抑制者；抗老化剂
diarrhea [ˌdaɪə'riə] *n.*	腹泻；痢疾
carvedilol [kɑːviːdɪ'lɒl] *n.*	［医］卡维地洛第三代 β 受体阻滞剂
bisoprolol [baɪ'sɒprɒlɒl] *n.*	［医］比索洛尔〈β 受体阻滞药〉
metoprolol [mɪ'tɑːprəlɒl] *n.*	［医］美托洛尔
angina [æn'dʒaɪnə] *n.*	心绞痛；咽峡炎；咽喉痛
diuretic [ˌdaɪju'retɪk] *n.*	［医］利尿剂
chlorothiazide [ˌklɔːrə(ʊ)'θaɪəzaɪd; 'klɒ-] *n.*	［医］氯噻嗪；氯噻（一种利尿降压剂）
indapamide [ɪndəpə'maɪd] *n.*	［医］吲达帕胺利尿降压药

hydrochlorothiazide [ˈhaɪdrəʊˌklɔːrəˈθaɪəzaɪd] *n.*	［医］氢氯噻嗪；二氢氯噻；双氢克尿噻
metolazone [ˈmiːtɔlæzəʊn] *n.*	［医］美托拉宗；甲苯喹唑磺胺
bumetanide [bʌmetəˈnɪd] *n.*	［医］丁脲胺；布美他尼
furosemide [fjuːˈrəʊsəmaɪd] *n.*	［医］呋喃苯胺酸；速尿灵（强效利尿剂）
torasemide [tərəˈsemaɪd] *n.*	［医］胺吡磺异丙脲；间甲苯胺吡啶璜酰异丙脲；托拉塞米
amiloride [əˈmɪlɑːraɪd] *n.*	［医］盐酸阿米洛利；氨氯吡脒
spironolactone [ˌspaɪrənə(ʊ)ˈlæktəʊn] *n.*	［医］安体舒通；螺内酯；螺旋内酯甾酮（一种利尿药）
triamterene [tˈrɪəmtəriːn] *n.*	［医］氨苯蝶啶；三氨蝶呤
clopidogrel [kˈləʊpɪdəgrəl] *n.*	［医］氯吡格雷（抑制血小板药物）；克拉匹多
coumadin [kəˈmædɪn] *n.*	［医］香豆素；香豆定：苄丙酮香豆素钠（sodium warfarin）制剂的商品名
hydralazine [haɪˈdræləzɪn] *n.*	［医］阿普利素灵，肼屈嗪
statins [sˈteɪtɪnz] *n.*	［医］他汀类药物
antiarrhythmic [ˌæntɪəˈrɪðmɪk] *n.*	［医］抗心律失常的，抗心律不齐的；抗心律失常药
rhythm [ˈrɪðəm] *n.*	［医］节律，规律；［乐］节拍；［艺］调和
amiodarone [ˌæmɪʊˈdærəʊn] *adj.*	胺碘酮的

TEXT B   Safe Medication Administration

Nurses spend a large amount of time administering medications for their patients. To ensure patients' safety, measures must be taken to properly administer medications and to minimize medication errors. Three checks and seven rights are the fundamental principles that nurses must uphold when administering medications.

Three Checks

To ensure the right medications are administered, nurses must perform three checks. Three checks in China refer to the checks just before, during and after drug preparation based on Chinese nursing practice standards. In the US, there have been the similar practice standards. Nurses are required to check the medication container label against the medication administration record (MAR) or computer printout three times: before removing the container from the supply drawer, when placing the drug in an administration cup/syringe, and just before administering the drug to the patient.

Seven Rights

The seven rights include the right patient, right bed number, right medication, right dose, right route, right concentration, and right time.

Right patient. Nurses must give the right medication to the right patient. To achieve this purpose, nurses need to check the patient's name whenever administering medications. In the US, nurses need to use at least two patient identifiers to ensure the right patient: asking the patient to state his/her name and normally his/her date of birth.

Right bed number. Nurses also need to check the patient's bed number if you practice nursing in China. It is important to remember that the patient's bed number may be changed during his/her hospitalization, so you need to check this with caution.

Right medication. An order is required for every medication nurses administer to a patient. A medication order could be hand written or the printout of the computerized physician order entry (CPOE) system depending on agency policy. CPOE allows the physician (or the nurse practitioner in the US) to electronically enter ordered medications, eliminating the need for written orders. Regardless of the type of order, nurses need to check orders at least three times when preparing medications and just before administrating medications.

Right dose. Medications should be given with right doses. To ensure the right doses, several principles should be observed such as: (1) when performing medication calculations or conversions, have another nurse or a pharmacist verify calculations; (2) when it is necessary to break a tablet, make sure the break is even; (3) when pouring liquid medication into a medication cup, hold the cup at eye level so you can accurately see the desired amount.

Right route. The physician's order needs to designate a route of administration. Always consult the physician if the route of administration is missing, or if the specified route is not the recommended one. When administering injections, it is important to prepare injections only from preparations designated for parenteral use. Medication companies label parenteral medications for "injectable use only".

Right concentration. The physician's order needs to specify drug concentrations for injections. Precautions are necessary to ensure that nurses give the medications correctly.

Right time. Physicians often give specific instructions about when to administer a medication. Nurses should administer the medication at right time. For example, a STAT medication should be given immediately after prescription; a medication ordered "after meals" should be given within half an hour after a meal, antibiotics should be administered on time around-the-clock to maintain therapeutic blood levels; and insulin should be given at a precise interval before a meal.

In the United States other rights have been added, for example right documentation, right reason, right response, right to know and right to refuse.

New Words

syringe [sɪˈrɪndʒ] *n.*	注射器
concentration [ˌkɒnsnˈtreɪʃn] *n.*	浓度，含量，专心，专注，集中，集结
print out [ˈprɪntaʊt] *n.*	（电脑）打印件
parenteral [pəˈrent(ə)r(ə)l] *adj.*	肠胃外的，不经肠的，非肠道的；注射用药物的
precaution [prɪˈkɔːʃn] *n.*	预防措施，预防，防备，警惕
antibiotic [ˌæntibaɪˈɒtɪk] *n./adj.*	抗生素；抗生的；抗菌的

Phrases and Expressions

around-the-clock	连续不断的，全天候的，日夜不停的
medication administration	给药

medication errors	用药差错
seven rights	七对
three checks	三查

FOLLOW–UP ACTIVITIES

Translation

A. Translate the following sentences into Chinese.

1. Nurses need to check the patient's name whenever administering medications so as to give the right medication to the right patient.

_____

_____

2. A medication order could be in the hand-written form or the print out of the computerized physician order entry system depending on agency policy.

_____

_____

3. When administering injections, it is important to prepare injections only from preparations designated for parenteral use.

_____

_____

4. Physicians often give specific instructions about when to administer a medication, so nurses should administer the medication at right time.

_____

_____

B. Translate the following paragraphs into English.

1. "三查" 是指操作前查、操作中查和操作后查。

_____

_____

2. "七对" 是指核对患者的姓名、床号、药名、每次剂量、给药方法、浓度和给药时间。

_____

_____

3. "三查七对" 是护士在给患者用药时必须执行的基本原则。

_____

_____

4. 为确保患者安全，必须采取措施正确用药，以降低用药差错。

_____

_____

Unit Seven
Specimen Collection

扫一扫，查阅本章数字资源，含PPT、音视频、图片等

After studying this unit, you are required to:

- master the basic procedures and rationales of specimen collection
- be able to communicate with a foreign patient to collect specimens in English
- acquire basic knowledge of HIV and learn to treat it

Part Ⅰ Listening & Speaking

Task 1 Video Watching

1. Watch the video and discuss the following questions in pairs.

1) Why is handwashing important before or after puncture?

2) What's the advantage of the straw for IV cannula compared with the needle?

3) Can you describe the equipment needed for an IV?

4) What's the possible diagnosis of the patient?

2. Linda, the ward nurse, is admitting Mrs. Johns. Listen to the conversation and answer the following questions.

1) Why does Mrs. Johns need oxygen therapy?

2) How does Linda identify the patient?

3) What's the difference in the oxygen level before and after the patient receives the oxygen?

4) When does Linda loosen the rubber band?

3. In pairs, discuss how you might change your approach to collect the following specimens.

1) a sputum culture specimen via tracheal intubation.

2) an arterial blood specimen.

Task 2 Dialogue

In pairs, practice the following dialogue and memorize the useful words and expressions.

COLLECTING SPECIMENS FOR A PATIENT

(N: Nurse   P: Patient)

N: Good morning, Mrs Zhao. I'm Wang Ping, the nurse on duty. Did you eat or drink anything this morning?

P: No, I didn't. I was told to fast after midnight for the blood test this morning.

N: Great. Thanks for your cooperation.

P: I'm very thirsty. I usually drink some water as soon as I wake up.

N: It'll be done very soon. Then you can have something to drink. Could I have your arm, please?

P: This one; but my veins don't stand out clearly.

N: I'll try to do it with great care, Mrs Zhao. Relax, please.

P: I'll try.

N: Now clench your fist, and don't look at it if you're nervous. Here, the needle is in.

P: How much blood do you need?

N: Take it easy, only 8 mL. You can unclench your hand now. Ok, it's done. Please press this area tightly with the cotton wool for a while to stop bleeding.

P: Is that all?

N: Yes, Mrs Zhao. The doctor has also ordered urine and stool specimens. Here are two containers with your name labels on them.

P: How can I collect the urine samples?

N: Put on this pair of disposable gloves and hold this little cup. After the stream of urine starts with good flow, place the cup under the stream. Pass some urine into the cup up to the 1/3 mark.

N: What about stool specimen?

N: Take a clean bedpan to the washroom. Pass your stool into the bedpan and collect a little lump of stool with this stick and put it in this paper box.

P: Where should I put the containers with specimens?

N: On the table just outside the washroom, please.

P: Got it, thank you.

N: You're welcome.

Part II Reading

Reading Guidance

As a qualified nurse, you are supposed to collect different specimens skillfully. The procedure and rationale should be followed when you are collecting specimens. In addition, specimens should be sent to the laboratory immediately and be placed in the proper place. If you are required to obtain blood samples of a client with HIV, it will be vital to refrain from occupational exposure.

Before Class

Please think carefully about these questions and discuss with your classmates.

- **Why should a sputum specimen be collected early in the morning?**

- **When nurses are collecting a throat culture, how can they avoid cross infection?**

- **What kind of tests are stool samples used for?**

TEXT A   Specimen Collection

One means of gathering information about the client's health status is by identifying pathogens and analyzing urine, blood, sputum, and feces. As a practical nurse, you may be in charge of collecting and labeling specimens for analysis and ensuring their delivery to the lab. Always wear gloves to protect yourself and prevent the spread of diseases whenever you work with body fluids. Washing hands carefully also helps prevent the spread of disease.

Throat Culture

Throat cultures are done to isolate and identify a bacterial or fungal infection in the throat. The slide or medium is incubated in the laboratory to determine which organism is the cause of a throat disorder. A sample of mucus and secretions is collected by swabbing the throat and placing the sample into a special cup that allows infection to grow. A determination of which drug is most effective against a particular organism may be also done. A full culture and sensitivity test takes several days because the organisms need time to grow. If strep infection is suspected, a quick strep test has to be done. Then antibiotic therapy can be started immediately.

Procedures for a Throat Culture

a. Wash hands and put on clean gloves to reduce transmission of microorganisms.

b. Use the flashlight to illuminate the back of the throat. Depress the anterior one third of the tongue with a tongue blade for better visualization.

c. Ask the patient to tilt the head backward, open the mouth wide and say "Ah". Swab the tonsillar area from side to side in a quick, gentle motion. Make sure that inflamed and purulent sites are included.

d. Withdraw the swab without touching the tongue, cheeks, or teeth to avoid erroneous culture results.

e. Place the cotton-tipped applicator into the culture tube immediately.

f. Label with the patient's name and ward number to prevent identification mistakes.

g. Discard the tongue depressor and remove gloves. Wash hands.

Sputum Specimen

Sputum is a thick fluid produced in the lungs and adjacent airways. Sampling may be performed by sputum being expectorated, induced or taken via an endotracheal tube with a protected specimen brush in an intensive care setting. Generally speaking, a sputum specimen should be collected early in the morning and taken for three consecutive days.

Procedures for Sputum Specimen

a. Wash hands and gather the equipment.

b. Provide privacy for the patient and explain the procedure. Place the tissues nearby and have the patient rinse his or her mouth with clear water to remove any food particles.

c. Assist the patient to a sitting position, have him take several deep breaths and then cough deeply to expectorate the sputum into the sterile container. Tell the patient to avoid touching the inside of the container.

d. Provide the patient with tissues to wipe his or her mouth.

e. Wash hands, label each specimen with the patient's name and complete the laboratory request form. Send the specimen to the laboratory immediately.

f. Record the amount, consistency, and color of the sputum collected, as well as the time and date in the nursing notes.

Stool Specimen

A stool specimen is often collected for blood, bacteria, ova and parasites tests. For instance, the fecal occult blood test that is useful in diagnosing gastric and intestinal irritation, GI bleeding, upper GI ulcers and colon cancer, detects microscopic amounts of blood in the stool. Tests performed by the laboratory for occult blood in the stool and stool cultures require only a small sample. Collect about 2.54 cm (1 inch) of formed stool or 15 to 30 mL of liquid diarrhea stool.

Procedures for Stool Specimen

a. Explain the purpose of the test and ways for the patient to assist.

b. Perform hand hygiene and put on disposable gloves when handling any bodily discharge.

c. Obtain a stool specimen from the patient, commode, specimen cup, or bedpan.

d. Use the tongue blade to transfer a portion of the feces to the specimen container.

e. Cover the container and label it with the patient's name.

f. Deliver the specimen to the lab immediately. Tests for parasites and ova require the stool to be warm.

g. If an infant's stool is to be examined, place the diaper in a leakproof bag, label it, and take the diaper and request form to the lab immediately.

Urine Specimen

A urinalysis is included in a health examination, and as part of the admission process for all inpatients. Simple urine tests, such as for sugar and acetone, are often performed by the nurse in the hospital. Urine is assessed first for its physical appearance:

a. Color. Urine varies in appearance, depending principally upon a body's level of hydration, as well as other factors. Normal urine is a transparent solution ranging from colorless to amber but is usually a pale yellow. Sometimes, urine color indicates possible underlying diseases. For instance, bloody urine, termed as hematuria, is a symptom of a wide variety of medical conditions. Dark orange to brown urine can be a symptom of jaundice, rhabdomyolysis or Gilbert's syndrome.

b. Odor. The odor of urine can reflect specific diseases. For example, an individual with diabetes mellitus may present a sweetened urine odor. This can be due to kidney diseases as well, such as kidney stones. When there is an infection in the urinary tract, the urine may take on a foul-smelling odor as well as appearing cloudy or bloody.

Midstream Urine Specimen

Midstream urine to be used for culture and sensitivity can be collected without using an invasive method such as catheterization. This procedure is best accomplished while the patient is urinating, on the toilet because the use of a urinal or bedpan increases the risk of contamination.

24-Hour Urine Specimen

A 24-hour urine collection always begins with an empty bladder so that the urine collected is not "left over" from previous hours. In addition, the container for collecting urine must be kept cool until the urine is taken to the lab.

Pregnancy Urine Test

Most pregnancy tests are based on the fact that the hormone human chorionic gonadotropin (HCG) is secreted by the chorionic villi of the placenta. This hormone is possible to be detected in small amounts.

New Words

pathogen ['pæθədʒən] *n.*	病菌；病原体
feces ['fi:si:z] *n.*	粪；屎；渣滓
incubate ['ɪŋkjubeɪt] *n.*	（卵）被孵化；逐渐形成；潜伏（在体内）
organism ['ɔ:gənɪzəm] *n.*	有机物，有机体；生物
tonsillar ['ta:nslə] *adj.*	扁桃体（腺）的
purulent ['pjʊərələnt] *adj.*	脓的；含脓的
respiratory ['respərətəri] *adj.*	呼吸的，呼吸用的
sterile ['steraɪl] *adj.*	不生育的，不能生殖的；无菌的，消过毒的
microscopic [ˌmaɪkrə'skɒpɪk] *adj.*	显微镜的，用显微镜可见的；微小的，细微的
hematuria [ˌhi:mə'tjʊərɪə] *n.*	血尿；血尿症
jaundice ['dʒɔ:ndɪs] *n.*	黄疸；偏见；乖僻；使患黄疸
catheterization [ˌkæθɪtəraɪ'zeɪʃən] *n.*	导管插入
bladder ['blædə(r)] *n.*	膀胱；囊；气泡；囊状物
pregnancy ['pregnənsi] *n.*	怀孕，妊娠
bowel ['baʊəl] *n.*	肠；内部，最深处
gastrointestinal [ˌgæstrəʊɪn'testɪnl] *adj.*	胃肠的
urinalysis [jʊrɪ'nælɪsɪs] *n.*	尿分析，验尿
placenta [plə'sentə] *n.*	胎盘

TEXT B   Occupational Exposure to HIV: Advice for Health Care Workers

How Can HIV Be Transmitted?

Blood, semen, vaginal secretions, vomitus, breast milk or pus from a person who is infected with HIV (human immunodeficiency virus) may contain HIV and cause infection. Therefore, activities like unprotected anal and vaginal sex, needlestick injuries or sharing needles are of great danger. Blood contains the highest concentration of the virus. However, "clear" body fluids such as tears, saliva, sweat, feces and urine contain little or no virus and do not transmit HIV unless they are contaminated with blood.

What Should I Do If I Think I Have Been Exposed?

If a skin puncture has occurred, induce bleeding at the puncture site by applying gentle pressure as you wash the area with soap and water. If skin or mucous membranes have been splashed by body fluid, immediately rinse the area thoroughly with water.

Get the name, address and phone number of the source person (client) and the name, address and phone number of the source person's attending physician. If you do not know the patient's HIV status, ask the attending physician for help. If you are at work, notify your supervisor. Do not waste too much time on details when in emergency and save the details later.

When Do I First Need to Get Medical Care?

Seek immediate assessment and treatment from your employee health unit, your private physician or the emergency department. If anti-HIV medication is indicated, it should be taken as soon as possible. If you have a skin puncture or cut, you might need a tetanus toxoid booster depending on the nature of the injury. Your physician will need to ask questions about the incident and other details in order to determine what treatment is necessary.

Should I Receive Post-exposure HIV Prophylaxis?

Post-exposure prophylaxis (PEP) involves taking anti-HIV medications within an hour of exposure. PEP, with the purpose of reducing the chance of becoming HIV positive, is a month-long course of emergency medication. If you think you were exposed to HIV, go immediately to a clinic or emergency room and ask for PEP.

Does Prophylactic Treatment Work?

Early post-exposure prophylaxis can reduce the risk of HIV infection tenfold. It is reported that early suppression of the virus can lower the "set point" for viral load and slow the course of HIV disease substantially. While there is compelling data to suggest the effectiveness of PEP, there have been failed cases. Generally speaking, failure has often been attributed to the delay in receiving treatment, the level of exposure, duration of treatment or all three.

Does the Treatment Have Side Effects?

Some of the medicines used can cause side effects. For example, zidovudine may cause headache, fatigue, insomnia and gastrointestinal symptoms (nausea, diarrhea, abdominal discomfort). In rare instances, lamivudine may cause pancreatitis and gastrointestinal symptoms. Indinavir and saquinavir may cause gastrointestinal upset and diarrhea. Indinavir has also been associated with kidney stones. Two quarts of fluid should be taken daily to reduce this risk.

How Can I Protect Others from Possible Exposure to HIV?

Until HIV infection is ruled out, you should avoid the exchange of body fluids during sex, postpone pregnancy, and refrain from blood or organ donation. If you are breastfeeding, your baby's doctor may ask you to switch to formula feeding.

When Should I Be Retested for HIV?

HIV testing may be repeated after 6 weeks, 3 months and 6 months. If you have not formed antibodies to HIV by 6 months, then infection did not occur. Until then, you should report and seek medical evaluation if you have any acute illness. An acute illness, especially if accompanied by fever, rash or swollen lymph nodes, may be a sign of HIV infection or another medical condition.

How Can I Cope with My Feelings?

It is natural to feel angry, anxious and depressed after occupational exposure to HIV. During the difficult time of prevention therapy and waiting, you may want to seek support from employee-assistance programs or local mental health professionals.

New Words

semen ['siːmən] *n.*	精液；精子
immunodeficiency [ˌɪmjuːnəʊdɪ'fɪʃnsi] *n.*	免疫缺陷
secretion [sɪ'kriːʃn] *n.*	分泌，分泌物；藏匿；隐藏
infection [ɪn'fekʃn] *n.*	感染；传染；影响；传染病
saliva [sə'laɪvə] *n.*	唾液，口水
mucous ['mjuːkəs] *adj.*	黏液的；分泌黏液的

prophylaxis [ˌprɒfəˈlæksɪs] *n.*	预防；预防法
zidovudine [zɪˈdovjuˌdin] *adj.*	齐多夫定；叠氮胸苷；叠氮胸腺
insomnia [ɪnˈsɒmnɪə] *n.*	失眠症，失眠

FOLLOW–UP ACTIVITIES

Translation

A.Translate the following sentences into Chinese.

1. If strep infection is suspected, a quick strep test has to be done. Then antibiotic therapy can be started immediately.

_____

_____

2. While there is compelling data to suggest the effectiveness of PEP (Post-exposure prophylaxis), there have been failed cases. Generally speaking, failure has often been attributed to the delay in receiving treatment, the level of exposure and the duration of treatment.

_____

_____

3. For instance, the fecal occult blood test, which is useful in diagnosing gastric and intestinal irritation, GI bleeding, upper GI ulcers and colon cancer, detects microscopic amounts of blood in the stool.

_____

_____

4. Until HIV infection is ruled out, you should avoid the exchange of body fluids during sex, postpone pregnancy, and refrain from blood or organ donation.

_____

_____

B. Translate the following sentences into English.

1. 基于你描述的症状，你需要做血常规、尿常规、大便常规等一系列化验。

_____

_____

2. 采集咽拭子标本时须在酒精灯火焰上消毒试管口，并将长棉签插入试管塞紧。若消毒不严格将会导致标本污染，影响检验结果。

_____

_____

3. 标本采集后应及时送检，不应放过久，以避免标本污染。

_____

_____

4. 血糖的检测可采用毛细血管采血法或者采集静脉血标本。

_____

_____

Unit Eight
Surgical Nursing

扫一扫，查阅本
章数字资源，含
PPT、音视频、
图片等

After studying this unit, you are required to:

● learn the importance of preoperative care

● know the job of a surgical nurse

● master what nurses should do before surgery

Part I Listening & Speaking

Task 1 Listening

1. Watch the video and discuss the following questions in pairs.

1) What do you think the nurse is doing?

2) What does a surgical nurse usually do while working?

3) Why is an operation a worrying event for most people?

4) What should the nurses do to reduce anxiety for the patients?

2. A nurse is visiting Mrs. Smith. Listen to the conversation and answer the following questions.

1) When will Mrs. Smith have surgery?

2) How will Mrs. Smith be carried to the operating room?

3) What kind of operation will Mrs. Smith undergo?

4) What will the nurse do during Mrs. Smith's surgery?

5) What measures will the medical staff take to alleviate the pain of the patient?

6) What did Jane, the Transport 1, ask Mrs. Smith to do?

3. In pairs, prepare a nurse-patient interview. Student A, a nurse, will insert a catheter into a patient's bladder and explain why she will do that and what the patient should do. Student B, a patient, will do as instructed.

4. In pairs, discuss how you can communicate with postoperative patients.

Task 2 Dialogue

In pairs, practice the following dialogue and remember the useful words and expressions.

PREPARING A CLIENT FOR SURGERY

(N: nurse   P: patient)

N: Good afternoon, Mr. McDonald. How are you feeling?

P: Good afternoon, Grace. I'm feeling ok.

N: Good. Do you know you're scheduled to have an operation tomorrow?

P: Yes, what time am I going to have it?

N: The operation starts at eight o'clock in the morning. You will get injections about 30 to 45 minutes before you leave for the surgery.

P: My wife wants to see me before my operation. Can she come here tomorrow morning?

N: Certainly she can. But she should be here by 7: 00am.

P: I see.

N: Did your doctor tell you what kind of operation you're going to have?

P: I'm going to have cholecystectomy.

N: All right. Have you signed the consent?

P: Yeah, here it is.

N: Do you understand the surgeon is going to do?

P: Yes, he was very thorough in his explanation. I don't have any questions.

N: Good! Then I would like to explain the preparation for the operation. If you have any question, please stop me.

P: Ok.

N: First, we'll prepare you by shaving and cleaning your abdomen. After shaving, we would like you to take a bath or shower.

P: Oh.

N: You're going to have a liquid meal for dinner. In the evening, I'll give you an enema. You should take in absolutely nothing by mouth after midnight.

P: I see.

N: You look worried. Do you have any concerns?

P: Grace, will this operation hurt a lot?

N: While there may be some pain, our goal is to manage it effectively. You're going to have general anesthesia. During the operation, you will not feel anything. We'll give you pain medication after the anesthesia wears off. Please make sure that we know if you are having pain, so we can make you feel more comfortable!

P: That sounds good. Thank you very much.

N: You're welcome. Please let me know if you need more information on your operation.

P: I will.

N: See you later.

P: See you.

Part II Reading

Reading Guidance

Preoperative preparation is vital to patient safety and thus it is a key nursing role. Patients who are physically and psychologically prepared for surgery tend to have better surgical outcomes. Preoperative teaching meets the patient's need for information regarding the surgical experience, which in turn may alleviate most of his or her fears.

Before Class

Please think carefully these questions and discuss with your classmates.

● **How important is the preoperative care?**

● **What preparations should the nurses make before surgery?**

● **How many factors contribute to patients' anxiety before undergoing surgery?**

TEXT A   Preoperative Care

Preoperative care is the preparation and management of a patient prior to surgery. Preoperative care involves many components, and may be done the day before surgery in the hospital, or during the weeks before surgery on an outpatient basis. Many surgical procedures are now performed in a day surgery setting, and the patient is never admitted to the hospital.

Physical Preparation

Physical preparation may consist of a complete medical history and physical exam, including the patient's surgical and anesthesia background. The patient should inform the physician and hospital staff if he or she has ever had an adverse reaction to anesthesia (such as anaphylactic shock), or if there is a family history of malignant hyperthermia. Laboratory tests may include complete blood count, electrolytes, prothrombin time, activated partial thromboplastin time, and urinalysis. The patient will most likely have an electrocardiogram (ECG) if he or she has a history of cardiac disease, or is over 50 years of age. A chest X-ray is done if the patient has a history of respiratory disease. Part of the preparation includes assessment for risk factors that might impair healing, such as nutritional deficiencies, steroiduse, radiation or chemotherapy, drug or alcohol abuse, or metabolic diseases such as diabetes. The patient should also provide a list of all medications, vitamins, and herbal or food supplements that he or she uses.

Bowel clearance may be ordered if the patient is having surgery of the lower gastrointestinal tract. The patient should start the bowel preparation early the evening before surgery to prevent interrupted sleep during the night. Some patients may benefit from a sleeping pill the night before surgery.

The night before surgery, skin preparation is often ordered, which can take the form of scrubbing with a special soap, or possibly hair removal from the surgical area. Shaving hair is no longer recommended because studies show that this practice may increase the chance of infection. Instead, adhesive barrier drapes can contain hair growth on the skin around the incision.

Psychological Preparation

Patients are often fearful or anxious about having surgery. It is often helpful for them to express their concerns to health care workers. This can be especially beneficial for patients who are critically ill, or who are having a high-risk procedure. The family needs to be included in psychological preoperative care. Pastoral care is usually offered in the hospital. If the patient has a fear of dying during surgery, this concern should be expressed, and the surgeon notified. In some cases, the procedure may be postponed until the patient feels more secure.

Patients and families who are prepared psychologically tend to cope better with the patient's postoperative course. Preparation leads to superior outcomes since the goals of recovery are known ahead of time, and the patient is able to manage postoperative pain more effectively.

Informed Consent

The patient's or guardian's written consent for the surgery is a vital portion of preoperative care. By law, the physician who will perform the procedure must explain the risks and benefits of the surgery, along with other treatment options. However, the nurse is often the person who actually witnesses the patient's signature on the consent form. It is important that the patient understands everything he or she has been told. Sometimes, patients are asked to explain what they told so that the health care professional can determine how much is understood.

Preoperative Teaching

Preoperative teaching includes instruction about the preoperative period, the surgery itself, and the postoperative period.

Instruction about the preoperative period deals primarily with the arrival time, where the patient should go on the day of surgery, and how to prepare for surgery. For example, patients should be told how long they should be NPO (nothing by mouth), which medications to take prior to surgery, and the medications that should be brought with them (such as inhalers for patients with asthma).

Instruction about the surgery itself includes informing the patient about what will be done during the surgery, and how long the procedure is expected to take. The patient should be told where the incision will be. Children having surgery should be allowed to "practice" on a doll or stuffed animal. It may be helpful to demonstrate procedures on the doll prior to performing them on the child. It is also important for family members (or other concerned parties) to know where to wait during surgery, when they can expect progress information, and how long it will be before they can see the patient.

Knowledge about what to expect during the postoperative period is one of the best ways to improve the patient's outcome. Instruction about expected activities can also increase compliance and help prevent complications. This includes the opportunity for the patient to practice coughing and deep breathing exercises, use an incentive spirometer, and practice splinting the incision. Additionally, the patient should be informed about early ambulation (getting out of bed). The patient should also be taught that the respiratory interventions decrease the occurrence of pneumonia, and that early leg exercises and ambulation decrease the risk of blood clots.

Patients hospitalized postoperatively should be informed about the tubes and equipment that they will have. These may include multiple intravenous lines, drainage tubes, dressings, and monitoring devices. In addition, they may have sequential compression stockings on their legs to prevent blood clots until they start ambulating.

Pain management is the primary concern for many patients having surgery. Preoperative instruction should include information about the pain management method that they will utilize postoperatively. Patients should be encouraged to ask for or take pain medication before the pain becomes unbearable, and should be taught how to rate their discomfort on a pain scale. If they will be using a patient-controlled analgesia pump, instruction should take place during the preoperative period. Use of alternative methods of pain control (distraction, imagery, positioning, medication meditation, music therapy) may also be presented.

Finally, the patient should understand long-term goals such as when he or she will be able to eat solid food, go home, drive a car, and return to work.

New Words

anesthesia [ˌænɪs'θiziə] *n.*	麻醉，麻木
anaphylactic [ˌænəfi'læktik] *adj.*	过敏性的；导致过敏的
malignant [mə'lɪgnənt] *adj.*	恶性的；有害的
electrolyte [ɪ'lɛktrəlaɪt] *n.*	电解液，电解质
prothrombin [prəʊ'θrombɪn] *n.*	凝血酶原
thromboplastin [ˌθrombə'plæstɪn] *n.*	促凝血酶原激酶
urinalysis [jʊərɪ'nælɪsɪs] *n.*	尿液分析
steroid ['stɪɛrɔɪd] *n.*	类固醇
metabolic [ˌmɛtə'bolɪk] *adj.*	新陈代谢的，代谢作用的，代谢的
pastoral ['pɑstərəl] *adj.*	牧人的；田园生活的；乡村的
asthma ['æsmə] *n.*	气喘，支气管哮喘
spirometer [ˌspaɪ'romɪtə-] *n.*	呼吸量计，肺活量计
splint [splɪnt] *n.*	夹板；薄木条
pneumonia [nju'məʊnɪə] *n.*	肺炎
analgesia ['ænəl'dʒiziə] *n.*	镇痛

TEXT B　Breathing Exercises After Surgery

Breathing exercises are encouraged after surgery to prevent respiratory complications. Breathing exercises include deep breathing and expansion breathing. Deep breathing exercises can enlarge the chest cavity, open alveoli, and expand the lungs, while expansion breathing exercises can strengthen accessory muscles.

Deep Breathing Exercises

The client should do deep breathing exercises every one to two hours for the first day or so after surgery. Deep breathing is done with the client in Fowler's position or in semi-Fowler's position after surgery. First, nurses should assist the client to a comfortable position and instruct him/her to place the palms of his/her hands across from each other, down and along lower borders of anterior rib cage and place the tips of third fingers lightly together. Then, nurses instruct the client to perform deep breathing according to the following steps:

1) Assist client getting into Fowler's position or semi-Fowler's position. Place the palms of the hands across from each other, down and along lower borders of anterior rib cage. Place the tips of third fingers lightly together.

2) Take a gentle breath through mouth and breathe out gently and completely.

3) Then take a slow, deep breath, inhaling through nose, and pushing the abdomen against the hands. (Tell the client he/she should feel middle fingers separate during inhalation and avoid using chest and shoulders while inhaling.)

4) Hold this breath to the count of three or five.

5) Exhale through mouth slowly as if blowing out a candle (pursed lips). (Tell the client that the middle fingertips will touch as chest wall contracts.)

6) Repeat the breathing exercises three to five times.

Nurses also encourage the client to take 10 slow, deep breaths every hour while awake during the postoperative period until mobile.

Incentive spirometry is often used to encourage the client to take deep breaths. Incentive spirometry can increase the flow of air into lungs to promote complete lung expansion. When using the incentive spirometer, the client must be able to seal the lips tightly around the mouthpiece, inhale spontaneously and maintain constant flow through the unit, and hold breath for 3 to 5 seconds when reaching maximal inspiration for effective lung expansion. The client may repeat this maneuver until goals are achieved. Usually, the number of breaths does not exceed 10 to 12 per session. The client should breathe normally for a short period between the 10 breaths on the incentive spirometer and end with two coughs after last 10 breaths.

Coughing and splinting may be performed along with deep breathing. Coughing can expel secretions, keep the lungs clear, allow full aeration, and prevent pneumonia and atelectasis. Coughing may be uncomfortable for the surgical client, but when done correctly, it should not cause injury to the incision. During coughing, splinting the incision area can provide support, promote a feeling of security, and reduce pain. A folded bath blanket or pillow is often used as a splint. The proper technique for splinting the incision site and coughing is described as follows:

1) Assume upright position, if incision is abdominal or thoracic, place one hand over incisional area and the other hand on top of the first; during breathing and coughing exercises, press gently against incision area to splint or support it; or place a pillow, towel, or folded blanket over the surgical incision and hold the item firmly in place.

2) Take two slow, deep breaths, inhaling through nose and exhaling through mouth.

3) Inhale deeply the third time and hold your breath to count of three. Cough to clear secretions from lungs for two or three consecutive coughs without inhaling between coughs, while firmly holding the pillow, towel, or folded blanket against the incision.

4) Cough two to three times every 2 hours while awake and examine sputum for consistency, odor, amount, and color changes.

Coughing is often contraindicated after brain, spinal, head, neck, eye or hernia repair surgery. The surgeon usually writes a "do not cough" prescription when routine coughing exercises should be avoided for a specific client.

Expansion Breathing Exercises

Expansion breathing exercises may be performed after surgery during chest physiotherapy (percussion, vibration, postural drainage) to help loosen secretions and maintain an adequate air exchange. Nurses should instruct the patient to do expansion breathing according to the following steps :

1) Find a comfortable upright position, with knees slightly bent. (Explain to the client that bending the knees decreases tension on the abdominal muscles and decreases respiratory resistance and discomfort.)

2) Place hands on each side of the lower rib cage, just above the waist.

3) Take a deep breath through nose, using shoulder muscles to expand the lower rib cage outward during inhalation.

4) Exhale, concentrating first on moving chest, then on moving lower ribs inward, while gently squeezing the rib cage and forcing air out of the base of lungs.

Breathing exercises are very important to prevent postoperative respiratory complications. Client education on breathing exercises is performed during the preoperative period. It is well recognized that teaching before surgery reduces apprehension and fear and increases cooperation and participation in care after surgery. The need to begin exercises early in the recovery phase should be stressed. Breathing exercises should be continued until the patient is up and walks regularly.

New Words

alveoli [æl'viəlai] *n.*	肺泡，泡，腺泡
incentive [ɪn'sɛntɪv] *adj.*	激励的，刺激的
spirometry [spai'rɔmitri] *n.*	呼吸量测定法
maneuver [mə'nuvɚ] *n.*	操作
aeration [ˌeə'reɪʃn] *n.*	通气，充气
atelectasis [ˌætɪ'lɛktəsɪs] *n.*	肺不张，肺膨胀不全
incision [ɪn'sɪʒn] *n.*	切口，刀口
thoracic [θo'ræsɪk] adj	胸的，胸廓的
contraindicate [ˌkɒntrə'ɪndɪkeɪt] *v.*	禁忌，显示不当
spinal ['spaɪnl] adj	脊髓的，脊柱的
hernia ['hɝnɪə] *n.*	疝，疝气
drainage ['dreɪnɪdʒ] *n.*	排水，引流，排水道

FOLLOW–UP ACTIVITIES

Translation

A. Translate the following sentences into Chinese.

1. Anxiety has physiological effects, which may result in hypertension, tachycardia and a rise in temperature.

_____

_____

2. Pain control is also an important concern. Near the end of surgery, the surgeon may inject a long-acting pain medicine at the site of the surgery to decrease pain for 6 to 12 hours after surgery.

_____

_____

3. Knowledge about what to expect during the postoperative period is one of the best ways to improve the patient's outcome. Instruction about expected activities can also increase compliance and help prevent complications. This includes the opportunity for the client to practice coughing and deep breathing exercises, and practice splinting the incision. Additionally, the client should be informed about

the importance of early ambulation.

_____

_____

4. Circulating nurses provide care to patients before surgery, which may include administering medications, placing IVs, performing preparatory procedures such as shaving and taking a thorough patient history.

_____

_____

B. Translate the following sentences into English.

1. 如果患者要做低位的胃肠道手术，术前需要清理肠道。肠道准备需要在手术前一天晚上早些时候进行，以免影响患者睡眠。

_____

_____

2. 许多因素会导致患者对接受手术产生焦虑，如对麻醉、手术过程及手术潜在结果等的担心。

_____

_____

3. 手术宣教包括告诉患者手术的开展方式、手术的预计时长，以及手术的切口部位。

_____

_____

4. 术后最常见的问题包括肺炎、出血、感染、手术部位血肿及麻醉反应。术后 48 小时内最常见的危险为出血及心肺问题。

_____

_____

Unit Nine
Emergency Nursing

After studying this unit, you are required to:

● master the basic cardiopulmonary resuscitation (CPR) techniques for adults

● know how to assess a trauma patient

Part Ⅰ Listening & Speaking

Task 1 Video Watching

1. Watch the video and discuss the following questions in pairs.

1) What do you think the nurse is doing when the patient is not doing well?

2) What information might a nurse need to collect in this situation?

3) Why is it important to assess the patient's signs and symptoms?

2. Listen to the conversation and answer the following questions.

1) What is the patient's problem?

2) Why does the nurse call for a rapid response?

3) What is the original diagnosis for the patient?

4) What might be helpful for the patient?

3. In pairs, prepare a nurse-patient dialogue. Student A, the nurse, is going to give the patient 20 mg of IV Lasix. Student B, the patient, has questions about this medicine.

4. Discuss in pairs about what else a nurse can do to help a patient with shortness of breath?

Task 2 Dialogue

In pairs, practice the following dialogue and remember the useful words and expressions.

AN EMERGENCY SCENE

(N: Nurse   P: Patient)

N: Hello, Mr. Benson? Can you open your eyes? Can you hear me?

P: Mmm.

N: Hello. Can you see me now? Don't worry, you're in the hospital. We're taking care of you. Your wife's here, too. Please nod your head if you can hear me. That's good. Well done. We're going to examine your chest and ask you some questions as we go along, ok? It's important for me to collect some information from you. Please respond to me with nodding your head or using your fingers if you cannot speak, ok? Please tell me what happened.

P: I thought I was having a heart attack. It felt like someone was standing on my chest. I had trouble in catching my breath. I was scared.

N: Did you take any medication? For example, aspirin?

P: Uh yes, I took two (holding up two fingers).

N: Two. Your wife told us that you've had angina. Did your doctor give you any nitroglycerine tablets to take in case you had chest pain?

P: Yes. But I couldn't find them.

N: You did the right thing for calling 120. We'll make sure everything is fine. We are going to do an ECG. Do you know what that is? It's a tracing of the electrical activity of your heart—so we can better understand why you had the pain.

N: What were you doing when you had the pain?

P: Oh, just doing some gardening around the house, some standing and bending over but nothing heavy.

N: I see. It's all right. Don't move please; lie as still as you can until we complete the ECG.

Part Ⅱ Reading

Reading Guidance

The American Heart Association is the nation's oldest and largest voluntary organization dedicated to fighting heart disease and stroke. The purpose of this Executive Summary is to provide an overview of the new or revised recommendations contained in the 2015 Guidelines Update. The AHA ECC Committee has set an impact goal of doubling bystander CPR rates and doubling cardiac arrest survival by 2020. Much work will be needed across the entire spectrum of knowledge translation to reach this important goal.

Before Class

Please think carefully about these questions and discuss with your classmates.

● **How important is the guideline for health care providers?**

● **How do you respond when finding a victim unresponsive?**

● **How can health care providers keep up-to-date with the revisions?**

TEXT A   2015 AHA CPR & ECC Guidelines

The publication of the 2015 American Heart Association (AHA) Guidelines Update for Cardiopulmonary Resuscitation (CPR) and Emergency Cardiovascular Care (ECC) marks 49 years since the first CPR guidelines were published in 1966 by an Ad Hoc Committee on Cardiopulmonary Resuscitation established by the National Academy of Sciences of the National Research Council. Since that time, periodic revisions to the Guidelines have been published by the AHA in 1974, 1980, 1986, 1992, 2000, 2005, 2010, and now 2015. The 2015 Guidelines Update marks the beginning of a new era for the AHA Guidelines for CPR and ECC, because the Guidelines will transition from a 5-year cycle of periodic revisions and updates to a Web-based format that is continuously updated. The 2010 AHA Guidelines for CPR and ECC provided a comprehensive review of evidence-based recommendations for resuscitation, ECC, and first aid. The 2015 AHA Guidelines Update for CPR and ECC focuses on topics with significant new science or ongoing controversy, and so serves as an update to the 2010 AHA Guidelines for CPR and ECC rather than a complete revision of the Guidelines.

Systems of Care and Continuous Quality Improvement

There have been several changes to the organization of the 2015 Guidelines Update compared with 2010. "Systems of Care and Continuous Quality Improvement" is an important new Part that focuses on the integrated structures and processes that are necessary to create systems of care for both in-hospital and out-of-hospital resuscitation capable of measuring and improving quality and patient outcomes. This Part replaces the "CPR Overview" Part of the 2010 Guidelines. The 2015 Guidelines Update provides stakeholders with a new perspective on systems of care, differentiating in-hospital cardiac arrests (IHCAs) from out-of-hospital cardiac arrests (OHCAs). Major highlights include:

● A universal taxonomy of systems of care.

● Separation of the AHA adult Chain of Survival into 2 chains: one for in-hospital and one for out-of-hospital systems of care.

● Review of best evidence on how these cardiac arrest systems of care are reviewed, with a focus on cardiac arrest, ST-segment elevation myocardial infarction (STEMI), and stroke.

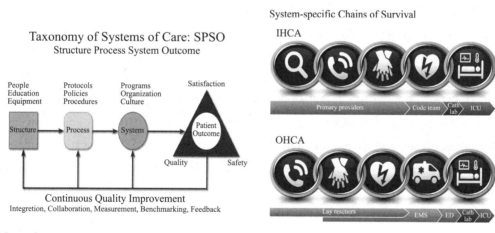

Education

Another new part of the 2015 Guidelines Update is "Education", which focuses on evidence-based recommendations to facilitate widespread, consistent, efficient and effective implementation of the AHA Guidelines for CPR and ECC into practice. These recommendations will target resuscitation education of both lay rescuers and healthcare providers. This part replaces the 2010 Part titled "Education, Implementation, and Teams."

Key recommendations and points of emphasis include the following:

● Use of a CPR feedback device is recommended to assist in learning the psychomotor skill of CPR. Devices that provide corrective feedback on performance are preferred over devices that provide only prompts (such as a metronome).

● The use of high-fidelity manikins is encouraged for programs that have the infrastructure, trained personnel, and resources to maintain the program. Standard manikins continue to be an appropriate choice for organizations that do not have this capacity.

● Basic Life Support (BLS) skills seem to be learned as easily through self-instruction (video or computer based) with hands-on practice as through traditional instructor-led courses.

● Although prior CPR training is not essential for potential rescuers to initiate CPR, training helps people to learn the skills and develop the confidence to provide CPR when encountering a cardiac arrest victim.

● To minimize the time to defibrillation for cardiac arrest victims, the deployment of an AED (automated external defibrillator) should not be limited to trained individuals (although training is still recommended).

● A combination of self-instruction and instructor-led courses with hands-on training can be considered as an alternative to traditional instructor-led courses for lay providers.

● Precourse preparation that includes review of appropriate content information, online/precourse testing, and/or practice of pertinent technical skills may optimize learning from adult and pediatric advanced life support courses.

● Given the importance of team dynamics in resuscitation, training with a focus on leadership and teamwork principles should be incorporated into advanced life support courses.

● Communities may consider training bystanders in compression-only CPR for adult OHCA as an alternative to training in conventional CPR.

● Two-year retraining cycles are not optimal. More-frequent training of basic and advanced life support skills may be helpful for providers who are likely to encounter a cardiac arrest.

Despite significant scientific advances in the care of cardiac arrest victims, there remains considerable variability in survival rates that cannot be attributed to patient characteristics alone. To optimize the likelihood that cardiac arrest victims receive the highest-quality evidence-based care, resuscitation education must use sound educational principles supported by empirical educational research to translate scientific knowledge into practice. While the 2010 AHA education guidelines included implementation and teams in its recommendations, the 2015 AHA education guidelines now focus strictly on education, with implementation and teams being included in other parts of the 2015 Guidelines Update.

Adult Basic Life Support and Cardiopulmonary Resuscitation Quality

Key issues and major changes in the 2015 Guidelines Update recommendations for healthcare physicians (HCPs) include the following:

● These recommendations allow flexiblility for activation of the emergency response system to better match the HCP's clinical setting.

● Trained rescuers are encouraged to simultaneously perform some steps (i.e., checking for breathing and pulse at the same time), in an effort to reduce the time to first chest compression.

● Integrated teams of highly trained rescuers may use a choreographed approach that accomplishes multiple steps and assessments simultaneously rather than the sequential manner used by individual rescuers (eg. one rescuer activates the emergency response system while another begins chest compressions, a third either provides ventilation or retrieves the bag-mask device for rescue breaths, and a fourth retrieves and sets up a defibrillator).

● Increased emphasis has been placed on high-quality CPR using performance targets (compressions of adequate rate and depth, allowing complete chest recoil between compressions, minimizing interruptions in compressions, and avoiding excessive ventilation).

● Compression rate is modified to a range of 100 to 120/min.

● Compression depth for adults is modified to at least 2 inches (5cm) but should not exceed 2.4 inches (6cm).

● To allow full chest wall recoil after each compression, rescuers must avoid leaning on the chest between compressions.

● Criteria for minimizing interruptions is clarified with a goal of chest compression fraction as high as possible, with a target of at least 60%.

● Where EMS systems have adopted bundles of care involving continuous chest compressions, the use of passive ventilation techniques may be considered as part of that bundle for victims of OHCA.

● For patients with ongoing CPR and an advanced airway in place, a simplified ventilation rate of 1 breath every 6 seconds (10 breaths per minute) is recommended.

These changes are designed to simplify training for HCPs and to continue to emphasize the need to provide early and high-quality CPR for victims of cardiac arrest.

New Words

resuscitation [rɪˌsʌsɪˈteɪʃn] *n.*	复苏；复兴；复活
controversy [ˈkɒntrəvɜːsi] *n.*	争论；论战；辩论
stakeholder [ˈsteɪkhəʊldə(r)] *n.*	利益相关者；赌金保管者
taxonomy [tækˈsɒnəmi] *n.*	分类学；分类法
prompts [prɒmpts] *n.*	［计］提示
manikin [ˈmænɪkɪn] *n.*	人体模型；侏儒
bystander [ˈbaɪstændə(r)] *n.*	旁观者，看热闹的人
choreograph [ˈkɒriəɡrɑːf] *vt.*	设计舞蹈动作；为……编舞
retrieve [rɪˈtriːv] *vt.*	恢复；重新得到
recoil [rɪˈkɔil] *n./vi*	畏缩；弹回；反作用

TEXT B Primary Survey of the Trauma Patient

The initial assessment of the trauma patient follows a protocol of primary survey, resuscitation (if needed), secondary survey, and either definitive treatment or transfer to an appropriate trauma center for definitive care. Absolute diagnostic certainty is not required to treat critical clinical conditions identified early in the process. When resources are limited (eg. one clinic), do not perform subsequent steps in the primary survey until after addressing life-threatening conditions in the earlier steps.

The primary survey identifies the life-threatening injuries and initiates stabilizing treatment in a rapidly efficient manner for the trauma patient. The steps of the primary survey are encapsulated by the mnemonic ABCDE (airway, breathing, circulation/hemorrhage, disability, and exposure/environment).

A-Airway Maintenance with Cervical Spine Protection

The first stage of the primary survey is to assess the airway. If the patient is able to talk, the airway is likely to be patent. If the patient is unconscious, he/she may not be able to maintain his/her own airway. The airway can be opened using a chin lift or jaw thrust. Airway adjuncts may be required. Suctioning may remove any debris that has accumulated in the oral cavity (blood, vomitus, secretions, etc.). In case of obstruction, an endotracheal tube should be inserted.

In addition, health care professionals should always assume that the patient has a cervical spine injury until it can be ruled out by X-ray films or computed tomography scan and clinical evaluation. All trauma patients should have a cervical collar and full immobilization in place to maintain the neck in a neutral, immobilized position until injuries can be ruled out.

B-Breathing and Ventilation

The nurse should assess breathing to determine patient ability to ventilate and oxygenate. Critical findings include the absence of spontaneous ventilation, absent or asymmetric breath sounds (consistent with either pneumothorax or endotracheal tube malposition), dyspnea, hyper-resonance or dullness to chest percussion (suggesting tension pneumothorax or hemothorax), and gross chest wall instability or defects that compromise ventilation (eg. flail chest, sucking chest wound). Pneumothorax, hemothorax, tension pneumothorax, and sucking chest wounds should be treated with a tube thoracostomy. Initial treatment for a flail chest is mechanical ventilation, which is also frequently required for other injuries.

C-Circulation and Hemorrhage Control

Hemorrhage is the predominant cause of preventable post injury deaths. Hypovolemic shock is caused by significant blood loss. Neck veins should be inspected for distension or collapse. Heart tones should be auscultated to make sure they are present, If external hemorrhage is identified it should be controlled by application of direct pressure or surgery. Hypovolemia, if present, should be treated by rapidly infusing a Lactated Ringers solution via 2 large-bore, peripheral, IV catheters, preferably placed in the upper extremities. If the patient does not improve, type-specific blood should be given. Cardiac tamponade should be treated by pericardiocentesis, followed immediately by surgery to explore and repair the source of bleeding.

D-Disability (Neurologic Evaluation)

During the primary survey a brief neurological examination should be completed to establish a baseline for subsequent assessments. A more in-depth exam can be done once the patient is hemodynamically stable.

The Glasgow Coma Scale is a quick method to determine the level of consciousness, and is predictive of patient outcome. An altered level of consciousness indicates the need for immediate reassessment of the patient's oxygenation, ventilation, and perfusion status. Hypoglycemia and drugs, including alcohol, may influence the level of consciousness. If these are excluded, changes in the level of consciousness should be considered to be due to traumatic brain injury until proven otherwise.

E-Exposure / Environmental Control

The patients must be exposed completely to have their injuries assessed thoroughly. Before that it is imperative to cover the patient with warm blankets to prevent hypothermia in the emergency department. Intravenous fluids should be warmed and a warm environment maintained. Patient privacy should be maintained.

After the primary survey has been completed and appropriate therapeutic interventions have been accomplished, the secondary survey can begin. At this time, all other injuries should be assessed by conducting a thorough head-to-toe examination, including a complete history and the reassessment of all vital signs. If at any time during the secondary survey the patient's condition deteriorates, another primary survey is carried out as a potential life threat may be present.

New Words

definitive [dɪˈfɪnətɪv] *adj.*	确定性的
encapsulate [inˈkæpsjuleit] *vt.*	封装
tamponade [ˌtæmpəˈneid] *n.*	填塞
hemorrhage [ˈhemərɪdʒ] *n.*	出血
debris [ˈdebriː] *n.*	碎片，残骸
cervical [ˈsəːvikl] *adj.*	颈的；子宫颈的
tomography [təˈmɒgrəfi] *n.*	X 线断层摄影术
immobilization [iˌməubəlaiˈzeiʃn] *n.*	固定
endotracheal [ˌendəuˈtreikiəl] *adj.*	气管内的
pneumothorax [ˌnjuːməuˈθɔːræks] *n.*	气胸
hemothorax [ˌhiːməˈθɔːræks] *n.*	血胸
thoracostomy [ˌθɔrəˈkɑstəmi] n	胸廓造口术
peripheral [pəˈrɪfərəl] adj	外围的；周边的
pericardiocentesis [ˈperiˌkɑːdiəusentiːsis] *n.*	心包穿刺术
hemodynamic [ˌhiːməudaiˈnæmik] *adj.*	血液动力学的
hypoglycemia [ˌhaipəuglaiˈsiːmiə] *n.*	低血糖症；血糖过低

FOLLOW–UP ACTIVITIES

Translation

A. Translate the following sentences into Chinese.

1. Hemorrhage is the predominant cause of preventable post-injury deaths. Hypovolemic shock is caused by significant blood loss.

_____

_____

2. Heart tones should be auscultated to make sure they are present. If external hemorrhage is identified it should be controlled by application of direct pressure or surgery.

_____

_____

3. The Guidelines will transition from a 5-year cycle of periodic revisions and updates to a web-based format that is continuously updated.

_____

_____

4. The clarified recommendation for chest compression depth for adults is at least 2 inches (5 cm) but not greater than 2.4 inches (6 cm).

_____

_____

B. Translate the following paragraphs into English.

1. 首次评估的目标是快速找出潜在的威胁生命和需要紧急处理的情况。

_____

_____

2. 大多数急诊医疗服务的目标或是为有紧急医疗护理需求的人士提供治疗，或是安排将患者及时转送到下一个特定诊疗机构。

_____

_____

3. 建议的胸外按压速率是 100 至 120 次 / 分钟（此前为至少 100 次 / 分钟）。

_____

_____

4. 将美国心脏学会（AHA）成人生存链分为两链：一链为院内救治体系，另一链为院外救治体系。

_____

_____

After studying this unit, you are required to:

● **master the basic process of a family visit to the local residents, especially the elderly people, the newborns and postpartum women**

● **be able to administer a family visit independently**

● **grasp basic writing skills for common documents which should be completed during family visit**

Part Ⅰ Listening & Speaking

Task 1 Listening

Listen to the conversation and answer the following questions:

1) What is home care?

2) What is the difference between home care and hospital care?

Task 2 Dialogue

In pairs, practice the following dialogue and remember the useful words and expressions.

VACCINATIONS

(N: Nurse   M: Mother)

N: Good morning, Madam. What can I do for you?

M: Good morning. My son is more than 3 months old. I'd like to know what vaccinations he should have.

N: You can start him on DPT vaccine.

M: What does DPT stand for?

N: DTP stands for diphtheria, pertussis and tetanus. All three vaccinations are given in one injection (shot).

M: If he gets the first shot today, when should I bring him back for the second one?

N: One month from now, and then one month later for the third shot.

M: Will there be any reaction after the shot?

N: Some children have a slight fever one or two days after the injection.

M: I see.

N: Has your son received the polio vaccine yet?

M: I am afraid not.

N: I will give him the polio vaccine today. There are three types. This red sugar pill is type I.

M: Can my son have polio vaccine and DTP at the same time?

N: Yes, he can.

M: When should I give the sugar pill to him?

N: The pill cannot be kept at room temperature. So you must give it to him as soon as you get home. Don't let him have any warm water or food until one hour after taking the pill.

M: Will there be any reaction?

N: No reaction in most cases. Come back one month from now for the sugar pill types II and III.

M: I see. Thank you for your help.

N: It's my pleasure.

Part II Reading

Reading Guidance

The family visit is an important part of home care for the residents in the community, especially for the elderly who live in their own home, women who have just given birth to babies, infants and children under 3 years old, and the disabled. Nurses provide health education and instruction during the family visit. This unit presents two examples of health education on diet and breast feeding which nurses frequently need to give during family visits.

Before Class

Please think carefully theses questions and discuss with your classmates.

- **How important is a healthy diet in our life?**

- **What nutrients are contained in breast milk?**

- **What benefits can the infants get from breast feeding?**

TEXT A　Healthy Eating

A healthy diet includes eating a variety of foods from the basic food groups: protein, such as meat, eggs, and legumes; dairy; fruits and vegetables; grains, such as breads and pasta; and fats and sweets. Simple as this may sound, it's not always easy to get the nutrition you need. You may eat more of your favorite foods from only one food group, and as a result, avoid others. Or perhaps you opt for convenience over quality when you are hungry.

A healthy diet requires some planning and purpose, and an effort to include a variety of foods in your meals. If you look closely at how you eat, you might find you aren't getting enough nutrients because you don't get the recommended number of servings from each food group.

So, it is important to pay attention to not only what you eat but also to what you are missing from your diet. To accomplish this, keep a food diary of everything you eat and drink for 1 week. Pay attention to serving sizes, and check to see if you are eating a variety of foods from each of the food groups. You don't need to meet the minimum number every day, but try to get the recommended intake on average over a week. You might find that making a few small changes will ensure that you're eating a healthy, balanced diet. Or, you may find that you are missing many important nutrients.

Once you are aware of nutrients that you may be missing in your diet or other ways that your eating is out of balance, you can begin to make a few small changes toward a more healthy diet. For example, simply adding a yogurt as a snack might be enough to meet your milk servings. Adding a sliced banana to your cereal will take care of a fruit serving.

Paying attention to serving sizes is also important. You may not know that a serving size of cereal is only 1 ounce (28 grams), which is 1/2 to 3/4 of a cup for most cereals. That means a typical bowl full of cereal is usually far more than a serving. So instead of a big bowl of cereal and milk for breakfast, have one serving (1 ounce) of cereal, and add a sliced banana and a small glass (1/2 cup) of juice. Use skim or soy milk instead of whole milk to reduce the amount of fat you take in.

If you find that you rarely eat fresh fruits or vegetables, make it a goal to include a serving or two at each meal. Only 1/2 cup of a cooked vegetable or 1 cup of salad greens counts as one serving. Drinking a small can of tomato juice, adding lettuce or bean sprouts to your sandwich, putting tomato sauce on your pasta—these are small ways to boost your vegetable servings. The new dietary guidelines recommend 2 cups of fruit and 2 and 1/2 cups of vegetable per day.

As you make changes, continue with your food diary. Set a weekly goal as you add or change what you are eating. For example, this week make it your goal to order a salad instead of French fries, add vegetables to your pizza, or bring a yogurt to work every day.

Just remember, food is one of life's greatest pleasures. All foods, if eaten in moderation, can be a part of a healthy diet. If your favorite foods are high in fat, salt, sugar, and calories, limit how often you eat them, eat smaller servings, or look for healthy substitutes. Your key to a healthy, balanced diet is moderation. Eat a wide variety of foods, especially those high in nutrients, such as whole grains, fruits, vegetables, low-fat dairy products, fish, lean meats, and poultry.

A healthy diet can actually help you lower your risk for disease.

To avoid disease, the 2005 Dietary Guidelines for Americans recommended eating a diet rich in fruits, vegetables, whole grains, and nonfat dairy products. The guidelines also emphasize watching calories to prevent weight gain, limiting alcohol, and cutting back on foods high in salt, saturated fat, trans fat, cholesterol, and added sugar. Activity is also an important part of the picture. The guidelines suggest 30 to 90 minutes of activity per day.

New Words

legume ['legjuːm; lɪ'gjuːm] *n.*	豆类；豆科植物；豆荚
pasta ['pæstə] *n.*	意大利面食；面团
yogurt ['jɒɡət] *n.*	酸奶酪；[食品] 酸乳
lettuce ['letɪs] *n.*	[园艺] 生菜；莴苣
boost [buːst] *vt.*	提高；促进；增加；改善
substitute ['sʌbstɪtjuːt] *n.*	替代品；代用品；代替者
poultry ['pəʊltri] *n.*	家禽；家禽肉

TEXT B　Breast Feeding

Milk from a healthy mother is the food of choice for a healthy infant. Breast feeding offers many advantages: nutritional, immunological, and psychological.

The infant receives immunoglobulins to protect against some infections. Human milk contains high levels of immunoglobulin A (IgA) and affords protection against several bacterial and viral diseases, especially those of the respiratory and gastrointestinal system.

The type of protein in breast milk is less likely to cause allergic reactions. Allergies develop in approximately 3 to 5 percent of infants fed on cow's milk formula. Because IgA prevents absorption of foreign molecules that might precipitate development of allergies, human milk will not cause allergies. This knowledge is of particular importance when there is a family history of allergies.

The nutrients in human milk best meet the infant's nutritional needs. Breast milk contains a high level of taurine, which is important for bile formation and brain development. The high level of lactose in breast milk may improve absorption of calcium, which is necessary for the development of bones and teeth. Lactose also promotes growth of the normal bacterial flora in the intestines. The majority of fat in breast milk is in the form of triglycerides, with higher amounts of several essential fatty acids. Cholesterol is also higher in breast milk than in cow's milk. The high level may be necessary to aid in the development of the central nervous system. Although iron in breast milk is lower than in formula, approximately 50 percent is absorbed, compared with only 7 percent of that in iron fortified formula. The increased absorption may be due to the higher lactose and vitamin C content in breast milk.

Breast milk is easily digested. Breast milk is more easily digested because of the higher ratio of whey to casein in human milk than in cow's milk (casein forms a large, insoluble curd that is harder to digest than the curd from whey). The enzymes that are present in breast milk also aid in digestion.

Breast milk is unlikely to be contaminated and the infant has fewer problems with over-feeding. Breast feeding is especially convenient for the parents as there is no need to prepare the bottles, no need to buy formulas and heat it.

Maternal organs return more quickly to their pre-pregnant condition. The balanced diet breast feeding mothers eat helps to improve healing.

The frequent, close contact between mother and infant may enhance bonding (initial attraction felt by the parent and infant). The frequent eye contact, skin to skin contact and sucking help mother and infant become acquainted and progress to develop feelings of love, concern, and deep devotion that last throughout life.

Both the mother and the infant must be positioned properly for optimum breast feeding. The nurse should make the mother as comfortable as possible before she begins to nurse. Pain or an awkward position may interfere with the let-down reflex and cause her to tire.

Before discharge, the infant should be feeding at least 10 minutes at each breast (5 minutes per breast for the first two days and 10 to 15 minutes on each side afterwards). The mother should be able to demonstrate the feeding techniques taught by the nurses and should voice satisfaction with breast feeding and confidence in her ability. This will be a major determinant of whether she will continue breast feeding once she is at home.

New Words

infant ['ɪnfənt] *n.*	婴儿；幼儿
breast [brest] *n.*	乳房；胸部
immunoglobulin [ˌɪmjʊnəʊ'glɒbjʊlɪn] *n.*	免疫球蛋白；免疫血球素
protein ['prəʊtiːn] *n.*	蛋白质
taurine ['tɔːriːn] *n.*	［化］牛磺酸，氨基乙磺酸
bile [baɪl] *n.*	胆汁
lactose ['læktəʊs] *n.*	［化］乳糖
intestine [ɪn'testɪn] *n.*	肠；肠管
triglyceride [traɪ'glɪsəraɪd] *n.*	［化］甘油三酯
cholesterol [kə'lestərɒl] *n.*	［生化］胆固醇
casein ['keɪsɪɪn] *n.*	［生化］酪蛋白；干酪素
maternal [mə'tɜːnl] *adj.*	母亲的；母性的；母系的

FOLLOW–UP ACTIVITIES

Translation

A. Translate the following sentences into Chinese.

1. You might find that making a few small changes will ensure that you're eating a healthy, balanced diet.

_____

_____

2. To avoid disease, the 2005 Dietary Guidelines for Americans recommended eating a diet rich in fruits, vegetables, whole grains, and non-fat dairy products.

_____

_____

3. Because IgA prevents absorption of foreign molecules that might precipitate development of allergies, human milk will not cause allergies.

_____

_____

4. Although iron in breast milk is lower than in formula, approximately 50 percent is absorbed, compared with only 7 percent of that in iron fortified formula.

_____

_____

B. Translate the following sentences into English.

1. 因牙齿不好而无法维持正常营养的患者会把改善营养不足作为健康护理的需要。

_____

_____

2. 维生素 D 在防治癌症和心脏病方面起着重要作用。

_____

_____

3. 有时人们不明白哪些食物是健康的，哪些食物可能对健康不利。

_____

_____

4. 产后护士的日常工作之一就是为其护理的母亲提供个性化的指导和支持。

_____

_____

Unit Eleven
Community Health Nursing

After studying this unit, you are required to：

● **master the special care needs of patients at different stages of the dementia progress**

● **pay attention to the caregivers for Alzheimer's patients, who face enormous pains and burdens, and to help families of the Alzheimer's patient obtain services they need**

● **learn the risk factors of the Alzheimer**

Part Ⅰ Listening & Speaking

Task 1 Listening

Listen to the conversation and answer the following questions:

1) What is Alzheimer's disease?

2) What are the signs of Alzheimer's disease?

3) What are the causes of Alzheimer's disease?

4) How to prevent the Alzheimer's disease?

Task 2 Dialogue

In pairs, practice the following dialogue and remember the useful words and expressions.

CONSTRUCT A HEALTH RECORD IN THE COMMUNITY

(N: Nurse   P: Patient)

N: Good morning, Mrs. Smith. My name is Mary and I'm a community health nurse.

P: What brings you here?

N: I'd like to ask you some questions for your health record. Do you have time?

P: Sure!

N: How old are you?

P: 48.

N: What's your occupation?

P: I'm a high school teacher.

N: Do you have any health problems now?

P: I have hypertension and type 2 diabetes.

N: Do you take medications?

P: Yes, I take antihypertensive and hypoglycemic drugs everyday.

N: Did you have any diseases before?

P: Yes, I had tuberculosis 10 years ago, but it has been cured.

N: Are you allergic to any medications?

P: Yes, I'm allergic to penicillin.

N: Are there any diseases in your family?

P: My father had Alzheimer's disease and my brother had diabetes. I heard that there is no known cure for Alzheimer's disease, and the treatment focused on alleviating symptoms and slowing down the course of the disease.

N: Yes, you are right. Alzheimer's disease is the only one we cannot prevent, cure or even slow down. I am sorry. And do you smoke or drink?

P: No.

N: Do you usually have a good appetite?

P: Yes, I do. I eat a lot, maybe too much. Ha-ha.

N: Do you exercise often?

P: Yes, I jog every morning.

N: Good! Do you sleep well or do you have difficulty sleeping?

P: Normally I sleep quite well.

N: That's great! Thank you for your cooperation, Mrs. Smith.

Part II Reading

Reading Guidance

Dementia is a syndrome in which there is deterioration in memory, thinking, behavior and the ability to perform daily activities. There is often a lack of awareness and understanding of dementia, resulting in stigmatization and barriers to diagnosis and care. Early intervention and appropriate use of supportive care by the community health nurse can be helpful to the cognitive and behavioral symptoms of the illness. The community health nurse should work closely with family caregivers, providing education and referrals when necessary to ensure the health and safety of their patients.

Before Class

Please think about these questions carefully and discuss with your classmates.

● **What is the nurse's role in caring for families with a dementia patient?**

● **How do the community health nurses support and assist the caregivers with an Alzheimer patient in a family?**

● **Why is it important for the nurse to help the patient and family identify community resources?**

TAXT A Dementia

Definitions of Dementia

Dementia is a syndrome—usually of a chronic or progressive nature—in which there is deterioration in cognitive function (i.e. the ability to process thought) beyond what might be expected from normal ageing. It affects memory, thinking, orientation, comprehension, calculation, learning capacity, language, and judgement. Consciousness is not affected. The impairment in cognitive function is commonly accompanied, and occasionally preceded, by deterioration in emotional control, social behaviour, or motivation.

Dementia is one of the major causes of disability and dependency among older people worldwide. It is overwhelming not only for the people who have it, but also for their caregivers and families. There is often a lack of awareness and understanding of dementia, resulting in stigmatization and barriers to diagnosis and care. The impact of dementia on caregivers, family and societies can be physical, psychological, social and economic.

Rates of Dementia

There are 47.5 million dementia patients worldwide, in which over half (58%) are living in the low- and middle-income countries. There are 7.7 million newly-diagnosed cases every year. In the general population, the estimated proportion of the general population aged 60 and over with dementia at a given time is between 5 to 8 per 100 people. The total number of people with dementia is expected to be 75.6 million in 2030 and almost tripled by 2050 to 135.5 million. Most of this increase is attributable to the rising numbers of people with dementia living in low- and middle-income countries.

Signs and Symptoms

Dementia affects each person in a different way, depending upon the impact of the disease and the person's personality before becoming ill. The signs and symptoms linked to dementia can be understood in three stages.

Mild or early-stage. This stage includes difficulty concentrating, decreased memory of recent events, and difficulties managing finances or traveling alone to new locations. People have trouble completing complex tasks efficiently or accurately and may be in denial about their symptoms. They may also start to be isolated from their family or friends, because socialization becomes difficult. At this stage, a physician can detect clear cognitive problems during a patient interview and exam.

Moderate or middle-stage. As dementia progresses to the middle stage, the signs and symptoms become clearer and more obvious. People in this stage have major memory deficiencies and need some assistance to complete their daily activities (dressing, bathing, preparing meals). Memory loss is more prominent and may include major relevant aspects of current lives; for example, people may not remember their address or phone number and may not know the time or day or where they are. They start to forget names of close family members and have little memory of recent events. Many people can remember only some details of earlier life. People at this stage require extensive assistance to carry out daily activities. They also have difficulty counting down from 10 and finishing tasks. Incontinence (loss of bladder or bowel control) is a problem in this stage. Personality changes, such as delusions (believing something to be true that is not), compulsions (repeating a simple behavior, such as cleaning), or anxiety and agitation may occur.

Severe or late-stage. The late stage of dementia is one of near total dependence and inactivity. Memory disturbances are serious and the physical signs and symptoms become more obvious. People in this stage become unaware of the time and place, having difficulty in recognizing relatives and friends, experiencing behavior changes that may escalate and even become aggressive. People in this stage have essentially no ability to speak or communicate. They require assistance with most activities (e.g., using the toilet, eating). They often lose psychomotor skills, for example, the ability to walk.

Strategies for the Community Health Nurse in Caring for Families with a Dementia Patient

Dementia is overwhelming for the families of affected people and for their caregivers. Physical, emotional and economic pressures can cause great stress to families and caregivers, and support is required from the health, social, financial and legal systems. Nurses who become partner with patients and their families provide nursing care by using a number of strategies in the community. The nurse's role should reflect the needs and resources of the patient and his or her family. Data from interviews conducted with nurses who provide care to people with a dementia patient illustrate the following guiding principles related to what care providers should do and not do:

● Don't assume anything. The nurse should collect data from the perspective of the person with a dementia.

● Adopt the patient's perspective. If the nurse operates from his or her agenda or personal cultural norms rather than from those of the patient, less productive and satisfactory outcomes will result. A good nurse-patient relationship is beneficial for both patients and nurses to establish trust in the nurse's work and increase patients' satisfaction. More importantly it improves the overall function of the system and the quality of nursing care, and benefits patients with comprehensive rehabilitation.

● Listen and learn from the patient. Gather data from the perspective of the patient and family. If the patient has severe memory deficiencies and cannot offer reliable information, ask the family or caregiver. Nurses must establish relationships that are beneficial to the patient's need and the family's need.

● Care for the patient and the family. The style and intent of patient and provider communication influences the acceptability of the interaction. A "conversational" style that establishes an equal partnership with the patient is preferable to an "open up the textbook" approach that tells the patient "here's what you need to do." The nurse should ask what the patient needs help with, what the patient would like to do, and how he or she can help.

● Be well informed about community resources. Learning about resources by reading a community manual is less helpful than meeting with the staff and agencies in person. People often respond differently to requests by someone they know and respect; therefore, it may be beneficial for the community health nurse to contact agency personnel about a patient and family need.

● Become a strong advocate. An important part of nurse role as care coordinator is comparable to that of a dementia advisor, whose responsibility is to act as advocate for the individual experiencing dementia; collaboration with other health and social care professionals and active development of these partnerships is essential in order to maximize the outcome for the person with dementia.

The community health nurse's perspective on dementia will influence the nursing role and the level of care he or she provides to people with dementia and their families. Whether or not the nurse chooses to work in a setting that specializes in health care services for people affected by dementia, dementia is a common disease that all practicing nurses will encounter.

New Words

dementia [dɪ'menʃə] *n.*	［医］痴呆
syndrome ['sɪndrəum] *n.*	综合征，综合症状，典型表现
deterioration [dɪˌtɪərɪə'reɪʃn] *n.*	恶化；退化；变坏，堕落
cognitive ['kɒgnətɪv] *adj.*	认知的；认识的
judgement ['dʒʌdʒmənt] *n.*	评价，判断；判决；意见；见识
consciousness ['kɒnʃəsnəs] *n.*	知觉；觉悟；意识，观念；感觉
overwhelming [ˌouvər'welmɪŋ] *adj.*	势不可挡的，压倒一切的；巨大的
stigmatization [ˌstɪgmətaɪ'zeɪʃn] *n.*	污名化；烙印化；描绘
prominent ['prɒmɪnənt] *adj.*	著名的；突出的，杰出的；突起的
delusion [dɪ'luːʒn] *n.*	妄想；错觉；欺骗；谬见
escalate ['eskəleɪt] *vt.*	使逐步升级，使逐步上升；乘自动梯上升
psychomotor [ˌsaɪkəu'məutə] *adj.*	精神运动的
conversational [ˌkɒnvə'seɪʃənl] *adj.*	会话的，谈话的；健谈的，善应酬的

TEXT B Alzheimer's Disease

Community health nursing is a synthesis of nursing practice and public health practice applied to promoting and preserving the health of the population. The practice is general and comprehensive. It is not limited to a particular age group or diagnosis and is continuing, not episodic. The dominant responsibility is to the population as a whole; nursing directed to individuals, families, or groups contributes to the health of the total population. Health promotion, health maintenance, health education and management, coordination, and continuity of care are utilized in a holistic approach to the management of the health care of individuals, families, and groups in the community.

Alzheimer's disease (AD) was named after Alois Alzheimer, a German doctor who in 1907 accurately described the typical brain alterations related to morphological, neurochemical, and physiological dysfunction. These alterations are irreversible. The cause is unknown; nevertheless, the latest research has enabled us to understand the molecular pathogenesis of the hallmarks of the disease in detail, i.e., plaques, which are composed of amyloid beta (Abeta), and tangles, composed of hyperphosphorylated tau. It is believed that AD is actually a group of related disorders distinguished by their symptoms, rate of progression, inheritance patterns, and age at onset. Researchers are exploring genetic and environmental causes, as well as defects in the immune system, as explanations for the disease. Until the cause is known, treatment can be only symptomatic.

Affected people manifest various stages as the disease progresses, from forgetfulness with long term and short term memory, to confusion and finally to dementia. These stages differ in length and intensity from one person to another. The symptoms include a decline in mental status involving changes in memory, language, praxis, mood, concentration, cooperation, thought process, and perception, with progressive deterioration. Mood changes occur until finally the person becomes completely passive. During the severe stages help is needed with the simplest activities of daily life, and the person commonly assumes the fetal position.

The onset of symptoms is usually noticed first by the affected person, family, friends, or peers at work, rather than by health care professionals. The person usually hides early symptoms such as memory loss and decreased mental ability, possibly for years. Progression is insidious, with a diagnosis frequently made more than 4 years after the onset of symptoms. The average duration of AD is 8.1 years, but duration is unpredictable: in some people the duration has been as long as 25 years. Victims usually die from another illness such as pneumonia, heart disease, or kidney failure.

AD causes mental anguish for the affected person. Caring for the individual places a constant burden on the families and caregivers. Community health nurses play a major role in helping afflicted persons and their families to obtain appropriate care. A mental health model that focuses on adapting to the individual's behavior appears to benefit the patient more than a medical model that focuses on correcting a disability. A specific pattern of care that emphasizes medical evaluation and drug management, combined with mental health care in nursing homes and day care centers that coordinate their services with social and aging services, is emerging.

A variety of social and aging services are frequently available in the community to assist demented persons and their families to improve the quality of their lives. Community health nurses are often in a unique position to help families obtain needed services. The Alzheimer's disease and Related Disorders Association (ADRDA) is a valuable resource for both health care professionals and clients. This association provides resource materials that help families to establish an effective management program at home, and offers group support services for families experiencing related stresses, and even assists families in identifying community resources skilled in working with affected persons. However, many health care services do not address the needs of individuals with dementia. Persons especially likely to be unable to obtain adequate services are those without families, individuals from minority and ethnic groups, individuals experiencing disease onset in middle age, individuals residing in rural areas, veterans, and the poor.

Support for informal caregivers is essential. The problems faced by families dealing with dementia are complex and stressful. Most of the caregivers face enormous pain and burden. The primary needs of informal caregivers are respite care, information on the diseases and care methods, information about services, and a broadened range of services. The range of services for persons with dementia and their families is very limited in many communities.

Community health nurses working with clients who have this diagnosis can find helpful resources and directions for research through published articles. An example of the material available to community health nurses working with Alzheimer's patients and their families in the home setting can be found in the August 1991 issue of the Journal of Home Health Care Practice. This journal provides the home health care professional with current information regarding the needs of the AD patient and caregivers, and includes assistance with nursing problems such as communication, nutrition, disorientation, ethical decisions, and respite for families.

New Words

morphological [ˌmɔːfə'lɒdʒɪkl] *adj.*	形态学的；形态的
neurochemical [ˌnjʊərəʊ'kemɪkəl] *n.*	影响神经系统的化学物质
dysfunction [dɪs'fʌŋkʃn] *n.*	机能障碍，机能失调
inheritance [ɪn'herɪtəns] *n.*	继承；遗传；遗产
praxis ['præksɪs] *n.*	行为；实践；习题
insidious [ɪn'sɪdiəs] *adj.*	阴险的；隐伏的，潜在的
anguish ['æŋgwɪʃ] *n.*	痛苦，苦恼；伤心，令人心酸
afflicted [ə'flɪktɪd] *vt.*	折磨；使受痛苦；使苦恼
veterans ['vetərənz] *n.*	退伍军人；经验丰富的人；老兵
respite ['respaɪt] *n.*	延期；（死刑）缓期执行；使休息
disorientation [dɪsˌɔːriən'teɪʃn] *n.*	方向障碍；迷惑
ethical ['eθɪkl] *adj.*	伦理学的；道德的，伦理的；凭处方出售的

FOLLOW–UP ACTIVITIES

Translation

A. Translate the following sentences into Chinese.

1. Dementia is a syndrome—usually of a chronic or progressive nature—in which there is deterioration in cognitive function (i.e. the ability to process thought) beyond what might be expected from normal aging.

_____

_____

2. Physical, emotional and economic pressures can cause great stress to families and caregivers, and support is required from the health, social, financial and legal systems.

_____

_____

3. Community health nursing is a synthesis of nursing practice and public health practice applied to promoting and preserving the health of population.

_____

_____

4. The problems faced by families dealing with dementia are complex and very stressful and place them at high risk for experiencing financial difficulties in addition to health problems.

_____

_____

B. Translate the following paragraphs into English.

1. 全世界有 4750 万人患有痴呆，超过一半（58%）的患者生活在中低收入国家。

_____

_____

2. 社区健康护士对痴呆的认识将影响护理的角色和提供给痴呆患者及其家庭的护理水平。

_____

_____

3. 阿尔茨海默病（AD）是德国医生阿尔茨海默在 1907 年首次发现并以他的名字命名，它准确描述了大脑在形态学、神经化学物质和生理机能失调等方面的典型性变化。

_____

_____

4. 症状包括精神状态的下降，如记忆、语言、行为、情绪、注意力、协调、思维过程的变化和知觉的进行性衰退。

_____

_____

Unit Twelve
Caring for Terminally Ⅲ Patients

扫一扫，查阅本章数字资源，含PPT、音视频、图片等

After studying this unit, you are required to:

● **master the basic knowledge of nursing for terminally ill patients**

● **discuss what services are provided by hospice care**

● **be able to comfort and soothe the dying people and their family**

Part Ⅰ Listening & Speaking

Task 1 Listening

1. Listen to the passage and discuss the following questions in pairs.

1) What does hospice care focus on?

2) Why is Faye and Wayne Payne's peaceful existence dashed?

3) What strategies does the hospice team use?

4) How does Faye Payne think about death after hospice care?

2. In pairs, discuss how you would like to spend the week if you had only a week to live.

Task 2 Dialogue

In Pairs, practice the following dialogue and remember the useful words and expressions.

A CONVERSATION WITH A CANCER PATIENT ABOUT PALLIATIVE CARE

(N: nurse   P: Patient)

Palliative care nurse Rose was having a conversation with Paul, a 40-year-old engineer with advanced stage cancer, encouraging him to talk about his feelings about his disease.

N: Are there things in particular that you worry about now?

P: Not really, I am sad at not seeing my daughter grow up, and at probably not being here long enough for her to have a memory of me.

P: I try to worry about things that are actually changeable. I worry about getting my book finished. I'd like to have that done to help my daughter to know me.

N: How are you now?

P: I'll give you my medical history in five sentences, if I can. I was diagnosed in Oct. 2012. At the time, I was having a lot of back pain, night sweats, and fever. I was diagnosed with lung cancer. I responded well to Tarceva (a chemotherapy drug) for about a year.

P: Then I had a relapse — last autumn, a course of chemotherapy, which was extremely difficult with a number of complications. Right now, I'm still kind of recovering from that cycle of chemotherapy. My last hospital visit was around Feb. 1st, my daughter's birthday.

N: (nodding) You went through what sounds like a grieving period, then threw yourself back into your life. What do you remember about getting hit with bad news a second time?

P: The idea that my life span was still going to be curtailed was always present in my mind. The hardest part is still thinking about how my wife, parents and siblings will react. I will have the easy part. I'll just be dead.

N: There is a quote that went something like: live each day as if it was your last. Take the time to do what you want to do if you want to write to your daughter or make a video.

P: Uh, I'll consider that.

N: If you need my help, please let me know.

P: Ok. Thank you. You are so kind.

N: You are welcome.

Part II Reading

Reading Guidance

If your beloved one has a terminal illness and all treatments have been applied, will you consider hospice or palliative care for him/her? Unlike other medical care, hospice care does not aim at curing the underlying disease but ensuring the quality of life as much as possible during the rest of the patient's life. This chapter will help you understand what hospice care and palliative care are, who provides hospice care and palliative care, when and where hospice care and palliative care are given and how they can provide comfort to the patients.

Before Class

Please think about theses questions carefully and discuss with your classmates.

• If your beloved one has an incurable illness and suffers from uncontrollable pain, what will you do?

• How much do you know about hospice care?

• Do you know the difference between hospice care and palliative care?

TEXT A Hospice Care

Patient S, a 70-year-old male, suffered from pancreatic cancer and cervical spondylosis with paralysis of both lower limbs as a complication. He had been repeatedly admitted for chemotherapy for his cancer, but the paralysis of his lower limbs gradually progressed, to the point that he needed to use a lift for bathing at home. He became completely bedridden and barely able to ingest food when his condition further deteriorated, but he chose to spend his remaining time at home and meet the end of his life there as he wished. In a sense, it is the role of hospice care to support him and his family by successful controlling of abdominal pain and helping him to live—and meet his end—with dignity.

Hospice care is a philosophy and a model for the care of terminally ill patients and their families. Originally, hospices were places of hospitality for the sick, wounded, or dying, as well as for travelers and pilgrims. In modern nursing, hospice is not a place but rather a patient- and family-centered approach to care. It was first developed in 1967 by Dame Cicely Saunders, who is best known for her role in the birth of the hospice movement, emphasizing the importance of palliative care for people dying from advanced cancer.

What

Hospice care is a formal system of interdisciplinary care for people who are nearing the end of life. By maximizing comfort for a terminally ill person, reducing pain and addressing physical, psychological, social and spiritual needs, hospice care has been shown to make people who have incurable illnesses feel better and live longer. To help families, hospice care also provides counseling, respite care and practical support.

Who and Whom

Hospice care isn't just for people who have cancer. Others who have heart disease, dementia, kidney failure or chronic obstructive pulmonary disease can receive hospice care. The hospice team includes physicians, nurses, home health aides, spiritual counselors, social workers, pharmacists, volunteers, bereavement counselors and other professionals, including speech, physical and occupational therapists, who can provide therapy, if needed. Enrolling in hospice care early might help you or your loved one develop a strong relationship with the hospice staff, who can help with preparation for end-of-life needs.

When

Hospice care is for a terminally ill person who's expected to have six months or less to live. This doesn't mean that hospice care will be provided only for six months, however. As long as the person's doctor and hospice care team certify that the condition remains life-limiting, and is willing to forgo curative treatments, he or she is eligible for the hospice program. Under Medicare, this decision includes what the patient is relinquishing.

Where

Hospice services are available in home, hospital, extended care, or nursing home settings. Many patients prefer to die at home in a familiar setting, whereas others fear burdening their families or prefer to die in a hospital or nursing home. It is important that the hospice team knows the patient's preference. When family issues complicate the options, hospice caregivers try to support the patient's wishes but also consider what is best for everyone. The following factors constitute the "requirements for good death," based on one's experience in home hospice care: (1) One's way of life; (2) One's relationship with family members (and others); (3) The receiving of optimal care; and (4) Peaceful death.

Keep in mind that no matter where hospice care is provided, sometimes it's necessary to be admitted to a hospital. For instance, the complexity and severity of patients' symptoms prevent them from being cared for at home; a hospital stay might be needed despite the willingness of family and friends to provide care.

How

People are never forced into hospice. Your medical team works aggressively to fight your illness and never pushes hospice when there are medical treatments available. Doctors tell you when it is unlikely that your cancer treatment is going to be successful, and doctors recommend hospice to patients, but it is always your choice about when and how to enter hospice treatment. By the time hospice becomes an option, hospice patients have experienced rounds of painful chemotherapy, radiation, surgery and other treatments and understand that it is time to end the fight.

By electing to forego extensive life-prolonging treatment, hospice patients can concentrate on their affairs in preparing for death: finalizing wills, saying goodbye to family members and taking care of any unfinished business. Hospice nurses, chaplains and other staff offer psychosocial care and expert symptom management, maintain a comfortable and peaceful environment, provide spiritual comfort and hope, protect against abandonment or isolation, answer questions about death, lead prayers and plan funerals or other arrangements.

Nurses especially can promote patients' self-esteem and dignity in several ways. The first is by giving importance to the things that a patient cares about—thus validating the person. Another way is by spending time with the patients as they share their life stories, helping them invest in and gain strength from their own meaning in life. The final ways are to call the patients by their surnames and titles, and to obtain their permission to include others in private conversations.

Hospice team members offer 24-hour accessibility and coordinate care between the home and inpatient setting. As death comes closer, a patient receiving home hospice care may enter the hospital for stabilization of symptoms or for caregiver respite. Hospice services facilitate mourning and provide bereavement visits made by the staff after the death of the patient to help the family move through the grieving process.

Human beings have the ability to meet their end, as well as to provide end-of-life care for others, and it is the role of hospice care to support persons in these situations. In a word, hospice stresses care over cure.

New Words

pancreatic [ˌpæŋkrɪˈætɪk] *adj.*	胰的；胰腺的
spondylosis [spɒndɪˈləʊsɪs] *n.*	椎关节强硬
paralysis [pəˈræləsɪs] *n.*	麻痹；无力；停顿
bedridden [ˈbedrɪdn] *adj.*	卧床不起的
hospice [ˈhɒspɪs] *n.*	收容所；旅客招待所；救济院
pilgrim [ˈpɪlɡrɪm] *n.*	朝圣者；漫游者
palliative [ˈpæliətɪv] *n.&adj.*	缓和剂；姑息的手段；缓和的
eligible [ˈelɪdʒəbl] *adj.*	合格的，合适的；符合条件的
forgo [fɔːˈɡəʊ] *v.*	放弃；停止；对……断念
relinquish [rɪˈlɪŋkwɪʃ] *vt.*	放弃；放手
chaplain [ˈtʃæplɪn] *n.*	牧师；专职教士
accessibility [əkˌsesəˈbɪləti] *n.*	可及性；易接近；可以得到
mourning [ˈmɔːnɪŋ] *n.*	哀痛；服丧
bereavement [bɪˈriːvmənt] *n.*	丧友，丧亲；丧失

TEXT B   Symptom Management in Palliative Care

Hospice care and palliative care are very similar when it comes to the most important issue of caring for dying people. In the United States and increasingly in most countries, palliative care and hospice have distinct meanings. Palliative care focuses on improving quality of life for persons of any age who are living with any serious illness and for their families. By treating pain, other symptoms, and psychological and spiritual distress, by using advanced communication skills to establish goals of care and help match treatments to those individualized goals, and by providing care coordination, palliative care is initiated at the time of diagnosis and is provided concordantly with all other disease-directed or curative treatments. In contrast, hospice care provides services to the dying in the last 6 months of life.

When providing care, both specific treatment for the illness and treatment to manage the multiple symptoms commonly experienced by chronically ill or dying patients remains a primary goal of palliative care nursing. Pain, agitation, dyspnea, respiratory tract secretions, nausea and vomiting are some of the most common potential problems that can arise in the last days and hours of a patient's life. Other disease symptoms which may occur, and may be mitigable to some extent, include cough, fatigue, fever, and in some cases bleeding.

Despite the availability of effective treatment options for pain, many patients suffer with avoidable pain at the end of life. Maintaining an ongoing assessment by frequently reassessing need for pain medication and other interventions is necessary. According to the analgesic ladder and repeat grading of the pain, opioids and non-opioid analgesics can be used. For example, non-opioid analgesics include paracetamol, aspirin and ibuprofen; opioid includes codeine for mild to moderate pain and morphine to treat moderate to severe pain. If the patient does not obtain relief from the prescribed regimen, nurses should advocate for change. Family members often worry about potential addiction to opioid medications. Not only is the incidence of true addiction very low, but a patient's need for pain relief at the end of life takes priority. But it is necessary to remain alert to the potential side effects of opioid administration: constipation, nausea, sedation, respiratory depression, or myoclonus.

Advancing disease pathology, anxiety, or delirium sometimes requires the use of higher doses or different drug therapies. Examples include the use of antipsychotic medications and anti-emetics to treat nausea and vomiting, benzodiazepines to treat delirium and morphine to treat dyspnea.

Routes of administration may differ from acute or chronic care, as many patients lose the ability to swallow. A common alternative route of administration is subcutaneous, as it is less traumatic and less difficult to maintain than intravenous medications. Other routes of administration include sublingual, intramuscular and transdermal. Medications are often managed at home by family or nursing support.

Although the palliative care teams have become very skillful in prescribing drugs for physical symptoms, and have been instrumental in showing how drugs can be used safely, some preventive interventions are recommended for all terminally ill patients. Preventive oral care is performed by using a soft toothbrush to gently brush teeth, tongue, palate and gums to remove debris, using diluted sodium bicarbonate (baking soda) or toothpaste and mouth rinse with diluted salt water after eating and at bedtime (usually 3-4 times daily). Prevention of bedsores is always better than cure. Nurses can instruct family to help the bedridden patient to move his or her body in bed or sit up in a chair from time to time if possible; to lift the sick person up the bed—do not drag as it breaks the skin; to change the sick person's position every one or two hours—using pillows or cushions to keep the position; to keep the bedding clean and dry and look for damaged skin on the back, shoulders and hips every day. Constipation is another common problem in terminally ill patients. Drinking often and eating any fruits, vegetables, porridge, and other locally available high-fiber foods are encouraged. Patients can take a tablespoon of vegetable oil before breakfast. If needed, gently put petroleum jelly or soapy solution into the rectum or administer a laxative such as senna.

Once the patient is near the end of life, comfort measures are recommended.

● Moisten lips, mouth, eyes.

● Keep the patient clean and dry and prepare for incontinence of bowel and bladder.

● Only give essential medications—pain relief, antidiarrheals, fever-reducing (paracetamol round-the-clock) etc.

● Control symptoms with medical treatment as needed to relieve suffering (including the use of antibiotics and antifungals, especially in HIV/AIDS).

● Eating less is OK.

● Skin care/turning every 2 hours or more frequently.

● Make sure pain is controlled.

Palliative pets can play a role in the end of life. For animal lovers approaching the end of life, contact with the familiar positive interactions with pets helps to normalise the hospice environment and reduce anxiety. Even for patients whose cognitive abilities have been hampered by illnesses such as Alzheimer's disease, clinical research has shown that the presence of a therapy dog enhanced nonverbal communication as shown by increases in looks, smiles, tactile contact and physical warmth.

New Words

sophisticated [səˈfɪstɪkeɪtɪd] *adj.*	复杂的；精致的；富有经验的
agitation [ˌædʒɪˈteɪʃn] *n.*	激动；易怒；烦乱
mitigable [ˈmɪtɪɡəbl] *adj.*	可缓和的；可减轻的
paracetamol [pærəˈsiːtəmɒl] *n.*	[药] 扑热息痛
addiction [əˈdɪkʃən] *n.*	上瘾，沉溺；癖嗜
myoclonus [ˌmaɪə(ʊ)ˈkləʊnəs] *n.*	肌阵挛
pathology [pəˈθɒlədʒi] *n.*	病理（学）
delirium [dɪˈlɪrɪəm] *n.*	谵妄；精神错乱；发狂
benzodiazepine [ˌbenzəʊdaɪˈeɪzɪpiːn] *n.*	苯二氮平类药物
dilute [daɪˈl(j)uːt] *adj.& v.*	稀释的，淡的；稀释，冲淡
bicarbonate [ˌbaɪˈkɑːbənət] *n.*	碳酸氢盐；重碳酸盐
rinse [rɪns] *v.&n.*	漱口；冲洗；漂净
normalise [ˈnɔːməlaɪz] *v.*	（使）正常化；（使）恢复友好状态
hamper [ˈhæmpə-] *vt.& n.*	妨碍；束缚；使困累；阻碍物

FOLLOW-UP ACTIVITIES

Translation

A. Translate the following sentences into Chinese.

1. Hospice care is a philosophy and a model for the care of terminally ill patients and their families.

_____

_____

2. By treating pain, other symptoms, and psychological and spiritual distress, by using advanced communication skills to establish goals of care and help match treatments to those individualized goals, and by providing care coordination, palliative care is initiated at the time of diagnosis and is provided concordantly with all other disease-directed or curative treatments.

_____

_____

3. As long as the person's doctor and hospice care team certify that the condition remains life-limiting, and is willing to forgo curative treatments, he or she is eligible for the hospice program.

_____

_____

4. Pain, agitation, dyspnea, respiratory tract secretions, nausea and vomiting are some of the most common potential problems that can arise in the last days and hours of a patient's life. Other disease symptoms which may occur, and may be mitigable to some extent, include cough, fatigue, fever, and in some cases bleeding.

_____

_____

B. Translate the following sentences into English.

1. 即使亲友愿意提供居家照护，有时患者病情的复杂性和严重性使得患者必须住院。

_____

2. 可将盐水稀释之后漱口或用 0.9% 的氯化钠溶液进行口腔护理，每天 3 ~ 4 次。

_____

3. 临终期间，患者肝肾功能减退，代谢和药物清除率下降，导致药物在体内蓄积引起毒性反应。

_____

4. 接受安宁照护（姑息护理）患者使用的常用药物包括：非阿片类或阿片类止痛药物以缓解疼痛，止吐药以缓解恶心，缓泻剂以治疗便秘以及镇静药以减轻谵妄和烦躁。

_____

_____

Unit Thirteen
Rehabilitation Nursing

After studying this unit, you are required to:

● master the basic knowledge of a stroke and stroke rehabilitation

● learn the basic techniques of stroke rehabilitation nursing

Part I Listening & Speaking

Task 1 Listening

Listen to the passage and answer the following questions:

1. What is a stroke?

2. What disabilities can result from a stroke?

3. What are the symptoms of a stroke?

4. What are the risk factors for stroke?

5. What can we do to prevent a stroke?

Task 2 Dialogue

In pairs, practice the following dialogue and remember the useful words and expressions.

POSTOPERATIVE REHABILITATION

(N: Nurse　　　P: Patient)

N: How are you? Did you sleep well last night?

P: Yes. I feel at ease after the surgery.

N: The surgery was very successful. From now on, the most important thing we should do is the functional training. I'll teach you every day. Please follow my instructions.

P: Thank you. I'll do my best.

N: OK, let's begin. Raise your arms and grasp the rings. You should do that at least 100 times every day. You may divide them into 4-5 sections.

P: OK. My arms feel so heavy.

N: You will have this feeling for the first several days, but you will feel the exercise is easier later.

P: I couldn't do it.

N: It looks like this exercise is too hard for you now, so let's change to another method. I will give you a small water bottle. Try to hold it and pass it between your two hands. Can you do that?

P: Oh, this is better.

N: Now, take a rest. I'll do some passive movement for your knees and ankles. The joints that you can't move by yourself will need this kind of passive movement. This exercise can keep the function of your knees and ankles.

P: OK, I'll do it frequently.

N: Now let me help you to do the toe exercise, try your best to extend the toes. Yes, very good, continue to move your toes like this.

P: Oh, my god, it almost requires all my strength.

N: But with your effort, the toes actually move. It's a good start. You have a great possibility of recovery if you persist. You are the most determined woman I have ever met.

P: Thank you very much. You give me the hope of recovery.

Part II Reading

Reading Guidance

Stroke knows no boundaries—every 2 seconds someone in the world has a stroke. Stroke damages parts of the brain that affect daily activities, like walking and talking. In this unit, we are going to introduce two types of stroke and the factors of successful rehabilitation. Especially, as a nurse, helping the stroke survivors and their families to help themselves is an important part of the nursing care. Rehabilitation nursing can help the stroke survivors relearn the skills they lose so that they can achieve an acceptable quality of life with dignity, self-respect, and independence.

Before Class
Please think carefully about these questions and discuss with your classmates.

● **What do you know about stroke and stroke rehabilitation?**

● **What can you do to help a patient recover from a stroke?**

● **What are the risk factors for stroke?**

TEXT A Stroke Rehabilitation

Stroke is a disease that affects the arteries leading to and within the brain. It is the No.5 cause of death and a leading cause of disability in the United States. A stroke occurs when a blood vessel that carries oxygen and nutrients to the brain is either blocked by a clot or bursts. When that happens, part of the brain cannot get the blood and oxygen it needs, so the brain cells die. The brain is an extremely complex organ that controls various body functions. If a stroke occurs and blood flow can't reach the region that controls a particular body function, that part of the body won't work as it should.

How the brain is affected depends on where the stroke occurs. It also depends on how much damage happens. The longer the brain goes without oxygen, the more damage there is. The two types of stroke are:

● Ischemic – A stroke caused by a clot blocking a blood vessel to the brain. This prevents the brain from getting the oxygen it needs. It is the most common type of stroke.

● Hemorrhagic – A stroke caused when a blood vessel to the brain bursts. This causes bleeding within the brain.

A transient ischemic attack (TIA), colloquially termed a "mini stroke", is a brief episode of neurological dysfunction caused by focal brain or retinal ischemia with clinical symptoms typically lasting less than 1 hour and without evidence of acute infarction. These patients are at greater risk for early ischemic stroke.

Stroke symptoms happen very fast. They may start, briefly go away, and then return. Remember, a stroke is a medical emergency. Every minute counts. You can recognize a stroke by asking 3 simple questions. Remember "S-T-R."

● S – Ask the person to SMILE.

● T – Ask the person to TALK or speak a simple sentence (clearly). Example: "It is sunny out today."

● R – Ask the person to RAISE both arms together.

If the person has trouble with any one of these three steps, call 911 right away.

Stroke rehabilitation can be an important part of recovery after a stroke. The goal of rehabilitation is to enable an individual who has experienced a stroke to reach the highest possible level of independence and be as productive as possible.

Rehabilitation is a dynamic, health-oriented process that assists an ill or a disabled person with achieving the greatest possible level of physical, mental, spiritual, social and economic functioning. The rehabilitation process helps the patient achieve an acceptable quality of life with dignity, self-respect, and independence and is designed for people with physical, mental or emotional disabilities. The process of rehabilitation can be viewed more appropriately as patient education rather than patient "care". During rehabilitation, the patient adjusts to the disability by learning how to use resources and to focus on existing abilities. Abilities, not disabilities, are emphasized.

Rehabilitation is an integral part of nursing. The principles of rehabilitation are basic to the care of all patients. The emphasis of rehabilitation is to restore the patients to independence or to the pre-illness or pre-injury level of functioning in as short a time as possible. If this is not possible, the aims of rehabilitation are maximal independence and the quality of life acceptable to the patient. Realistic goals based on individual patient assessment are established with the patient to guide the rehabilitation program.

The most important contributions to patients' rehabilitation are made by the patients themselves. Regardless of the severity of the disability or the skill of the rehabilitation team, the patient's motivation greatly influences the final outcome.

Successful rehabilitation depends on:

● Amount of damage to the brain.

● Skill on the part of the rehabilitation team.

● Cooperation of family and friends. Caring family/friends can be one of the most important factors in rehabilitation.

● Timing of rehabilitation– the earlier it begins the more likely survivors are to regain lost abilities and skills.

Rehabilitation after stroke can preserve or improve range of motion, muscle strength, bowel and bladder function, and functional and cognitive abilities. It includes physical therapy, occupational therapy, speech therapy, and swallowing therapy. Stroke rehabilitation nursing aims to:

- Aid physical recovery from stroke.
- Facilitate independence in activities of daily living.
- Reduce the risk of secondary complications and related conditions.
- Promote holistic adaptation to stroke-related disability.

As a nurse, helping the stroke survivors and their families to help themselves is an important part of the nursing care. Nurses who work with the stroke-survivors have two major responsibilities: to see that damage from stroke is limited as much as possible and to see that a rehabilitation program is planned and implemented.

Stroke damages parts of the brain that affect everyday activities, like walking and talking. Rehabilitation nursing can help them relearn these skills:

- Personal care activities, such as bathing, dressing, grooming and feeding.
- Speech and language problems.
- Interacting with others.
- Memory and problem solving.
- Walking and transferring, such as moving from bed to chair.

People who have had a stroke are at an increased risk of having another one, especially during the first year following the original stroke. Although some risk factors for stroke cannot be changed, others such as high blood pressure and smoking can be altered. Patients and families should seek guidance from their physicians about lifestyle changes to help prevent another stroke.

Because stroke survivors often have complex rehabilitation needs, progress and recovery are unique for each person. Although a majority of functional abilities may be restored soon after a stroke, recovery is an ongoing process. People who have had a stroke need support and encouragement from family and friends.

New Words

stroke [strəʊk] *n.*	中风
clot [klɒt] *n.*	凝块
ischemic [ɪsˈkimɪk] *adj.*	缺血性的
retinal [ˈretɪnl] *adj.*	视网膜的
dynamic [daɪˈnæmɪk] *adj.*	动态的；有活力的
oriented [ˈɔːrɪentɪd] *adj.*	导向的；定向的；以……为方向的
integral [ˈɪntɪgrəl] *adj.*	完整的；不可或缺的
ongoing [ˈɒngəʊɪŋ] *adj.*	不间断的；进行的

TEXT B   Mom's Stroke Inspires NBA Star

Before Paul George was a two-time NBA All-Star, before he was a player on the Indiana Pacers, before he was the tenth player picked in the NBA draft or led his high school basketball team to a league championship, he was the 6-year-old son of a stroke survivor. His mother Paulette's stroke at age 37 would change his life forever.

Mother Paulette's Stroke

"I was perfectly healthy, I never had high blood pressure or high cholesterol." Paulette said in an interview with the American Heart Association/American Stroke Association. Then one night there were hours of vomiting and a terrible headache before her twin sister called an ambulance to take her to the hospital. But all the lab work showed was a virus and she was sent home. Once home, things turned chaotic as she lost her vision. Then there was a tingling sensation that started in her toes and moved up her legs. Two days later, she was in the hospital again completely paralyzed. Confused over the source of her problems, a doctor gave her less than 24 hours to live. Eventually, doctors discovered the culprit: stroke, but no specific cause was ever determined. Everything changed after she returned home from the hospital and rehab. "I could look at people, but that was the most I could do. I lost everything." she said. Paulette had been a stay-at-home mom who had walked her children to school every day, but she was now confined to the hospital bed in her bedroom at home for nearly two years.

Long and Slow Recovery Process

Their house in Palmdale, California, became like a hospital room, with a wheelchair, bed and commode chair. Paulette couldn't speak or do much for herself, yet being home-surrounded by family made her feel safe and helped her heal. Portala and Teiosha did much of the household work. Eating dinner at the table, seated in her wheelchair and using her one good hand, was a milestone. Ditching the wheelchair for a walking cane was even bigger. "Happiness is medicine, too." she said.

The Encouragement from Mom's Stroke

He did well enough in his freshman season to be named to Sports Illustrated list of the most entertaining players at the start of his sophomore season. At age 19, at the end of that season and barely five years after he'd started playing basketball, Paul announced that he would enter the NBA draft in 2010. The Indiana Pacers drafted him with the tenth overall pick. A sports pundit at the time prophesied that Paul would eventually be the best known player from the 2010 draft. Although at the time he was not considered an impact player, he was a starter by his second season. "I've always been underrated, and that always drove me to stay in the gym, to work hard and to continue to push myself the same way my mom had to fight through her adversity, Whenever I feel like I've had a bad day, I think about my mom and it strengthens me. I've got to keep going hard for my mom." he said. His aptitude for hard work has paid off: In the 2012-2013 season he was named Most Improved Player in the NBA. He signed a new contract and was named to the East All-Stars for the 2013-2014 season.

To Do Something Big

With his career taking off, 24-year-old Paul is eager to share his fame with his mom, giving her a larger platform to spread awareness on how to prevent and beat stroke. That's what led them to the American Heart Association/American Stroke Association. "She always tells me that she really would love to do something big, and I want to make it happen." Paul said. "Telling her testimony of what she's been through is really her passion. I feel like she was put in a position to be able to use her voice, and I want to be an extension of her voice to really get that out there."

"It's been depressing and emotional, because I can't do the things I used to do and I'm not the way I used to be." Paulette said. "But I've learned my limitations. I know what I can do, what I can take, my exhaustion level. I try to deal with life as it is. I have that will to fight. The harder you work, the better it gets. The happiest part of all is that we're always together as a family — and that I'm still here and blessed to enjoy all that." she said.

New Words

chaotic [keɪˈɒtɪk] *adj.*	混沌的；混乱的，无秩序的
vision [ˈvɪʒn] *n.*	视力
paralyzed [ˈpærəˌlaɪzd] *adj.*	瘫痪的
culprit [ˈkʌlprɪt] *n.*	问题的起因；罪犯；元凶
commode [kəˈməʊd] *n.*	便桶
milestone [ˈmaɪlstəʊn] *n.*	里程碑；划时代的事件
gym [dʒɪm] *n.*	健身房
adversity [ədˈvɜːsəti] *n.*	逆境
testimony [ˈtestɪməni] *n.*	证词；证言

FOLLOW–UP ACTIVITIES

Translation

A. Translate the following sentences into Chinese.

1. Rehabilitation is a dynamic, health-oriented process that assists an ill or a disabled person to achieve the greatest possible level of physical, mental, spiritual, social and economic functioning.

_____

_____

2. The goal of rehabilitation is to enable an individual who has experienced a stroke to reach the highest possible level of independence and be as productive as possible.

_____

_____

3. Nurses who work with the stroke survivors have two major responsibilities: to see that damage from stroke is limited as much as possible and to see that a rehabilitation program is planned and implemented.

_____

_____

4. Because stroke survivors often have complex rehabilitation needs, progress and recovery are unique for each person.

_____

_____

B. Translate the following sentences into English.

1. 在康复中使用哪种治疗和服务取决于个人的需要。

_____

_____

2. 护士的责任是根据患者目标，密切参与患者康复计划的制订与实施。

_____

_____

3. 尽管康复类型、水平和目标有所不同，但康复的需求贯穿于各个年龄段。

_____

_____

4. 随着危重患者和伤残患者救治技术的不断提高，需要康复服务的人比以往任何时候都多。

_____

_____

扫一扫，查阅本章数字资源，含PPT、音视频、图片等

After studying this unit, you are required to:

● **be familiar with the origin and general history of TCM**

● **be familiar with the basic theories of TCM**

● **introduce the different forms of TCM**

● **explain the ways of performing acupuncture, moxibustion and** *tuina*

Part I Listening & Speaking

Task 1 Listening

Listen to the passage and answer the following questions.

1. What are the nutrients in food essential for?

2. How will people benefit from eating a variety of foods?

3. What do fruits and vegetables contain?

4. What role does fiber play in the digestive system?

5. Why do older adults need to drink water before feeling thirsty?

6. What have green tea and its extracts been used for?

7. What will be the consequence of skipping meals?

8. Why are processed foods harmful to health?

Task 2 Dialogue

In pairs, practice the following dialogue and remember the useful words and expressions.

COLD DUE TO WIND-COLD

(N: Nurse   P: Patient)

A patient, who is suffering from a severe cold due to wind-cold, comes to the hospital for help. The nurse on duty is asking him about the cold and offering some advice.

N: Good morning. You are a new patient. What is the problem?

P: I've got a bad cold.

N: How do you feel in general?

P: I feel cold all over, and have to wrap myself with a thick quilt when I am sleeping.

N: It seems that the wind-cold evil has restrained the defensive-qi in your body. Are you sweating at present?

P: No, I am not.

N: No sweating implies that the striae of skin and muscles are closed by the pathogen, so the sweat has to stay inside the body.

P: My joints hurt very much, and my neck can't turn around flexibly.

N: That is caused by cold pathogen obstructing the flow of *qi* in the meridians. Are you coughing?

P: Yes, I cough badly at night.

N: The cough shows the pathogen has disturbed the function of your lungs. Is there any sputum?

P: Just a little. It is white and a little bit yellow, and it is quite sticky.

N: The white and yellow sputum implies that the wind-cold pathogen has impaired the dispersing and descending function of your lungs. How about your appetite?

P: I had no appetite for the last two days.

N: Loss of appetite indicates that the function of spleen and stomach has been impaired. How about your bowel movements and urination?

P: I feel they are normal, as usual.

N: Have you taken any medication?

P: Yeah, I took some antibiotics, but they didn't work.

N: Well, let me feel your pulse and look at your tongue. The pulse is floating, and your tongue is pale with a thin coating. You'd better take some herbal drugs with pungent taste and warm nature to dispel the exterior evil. The Chinese medicine clinic is on the second floor. This way, please.

P: All right. Thank you very much.

N: You are welcome!

Part II Reading

Reading Guidance

What is Traditional Chinese Medicine (TCM)? How much do you know about it? In fact, TCM, a tradition for more than 2000 years in China, generates various clinical forms based on the same theories, among which, acupuncture, moxibustion, and *tuina* are widely accepted and practiced in western countries. This unit focuses on the basic theories, classics, and different clinical forms of TCM.

Before Class

Please think carefully about these questions and discuss with your classmates.

● **What is the core belief of TCM?**

● **What techniques can be employed to manipulate *qi*?**

● **What are the main functions of acupuncture, moxibustion and *tuina*?**

● **How can you perform acupuncture, moxibustion and *tuina*?**

TEXT A   Traditional Chinese Medicine

In the west, "medicine" is regarded as a way of dealing with illness and disease. In contrast, Traditional Chinese Medicine (TCM) focuses on achieving health and well-being through the cultivation of harmony within our lives. TCM is based on the Chinese concept of "*qi*" and the theory of "*yin*" and "*yang*". It believes that harmony brings health, well-being, and sustainability, while disharmony leads to illness, disease, and collapse.

The TCM Perspective

In the simplest terms possible, TCM is a way of looking at ourselves and our world that sees everything as a whole and considers everything in context. In TCM this perspective is called "holism."

This perspective is applied to everything affecting our health and well-being, from our diet, exercise and how we handle stress, to how we interact with our family and friends, our community and our environment. Thus TCM not only identifies and treats illness and prevents disease but, just as importantly, optimizes health, well-being, and sustainability in our lives and in our world.

Origin of TCM

TCM is a direct descendent of one of the oldest continuously practiced systems of medicine in the world, and can trace its roots back 2500 years. Since its inception, Chinese medicine has evolved through meticulous observation of nature, the cosmos, and the human body, and has developed into a very sophisticated and rational system of medicine influencing and being influenced by the many cultures and systems of medicine it has come into contact with along the way.

Today Chinese medicine continues to develop in new and exciting ways and is utilized by millions of people around the world.

The Most Influential Texts

Huangdi Neijing (*Yellow Emperor's Inner Canon*) has been the most influential treatise for more than 2,000 years. The multi-volume treatise presents views on the function of the human body and the physical world that remain the basic ideas believed by traditional medicine practitioners. *Yin* and *yang* are described, and so are the Five Phases of nature (wood, fire, earth, metal, water) and *qi*. It isn't known how or where these ideas originated.

Bencao Gangmu (*Compendium of Materia Medica*) is the most important traditional work on herbs and drugs. It was written in the middle of the Ming Dynasty era (1368-1644) by Li Shizhen (1518–1593), who was a doctor and a former official of the Imperial Medical Bureau of the Ming Empire. This text is usually called *Materia Medica* in English. The extraordinarily long and detailed tome was considered to be the most exhaustive and detailed text on traditional herbal medicine. It classified and described hundreds of kinds of herbs, medicinal minerals and medicinal animal parts. The *Bencao Gangmu* is considered to be the greatest scientific achievement of the Ming Dynasty. The treatise shows the state of Chinese medical theory before the introduction of Western medicine in the 1800s.

The *Yin-yang* Balance

The core belief of TCM is about the *yin-yang qi* balance in the body and its organs. Most TCM practitioners think that there are many kinds of *qi*, and the most basic are *yin qi* and *yang qi*. Everything is a balance between *yin* and *yang*. *Yin* is female, dark and tangible. *Yang* is male, light, and intangible. Females have more *yin qi*, and males have more *yang qi*, and as people age, they lose *qi*.

The *qi* is life energy, and its flow in the body depends on the environment and what happens to the body. The balance of *qi* in the parts of the body depends on the flow of various kinds of *qi* and fluids. Injury, physical suffering, and lack of proper food cause a *qi* deficiency.

The core idea of TCM is that people can increase or decrease various *qi* in the body and its parts by different medical techniques to create a healthful *yin-yang* balance. Each person and each part of the body has an ideal point of balance of *yin* and *yang* for optimal health. Some techniques are more appropriate for increasing *yang qi*, and some are appropriate for decreasing *yang qi*, and likewise for *yin qi*.

Various Techniques That Manipulate Various *Qi*

Qi deficiencies in a person or a body part can be corrected by eating proper food, taking herbs and medicines, using physical manipulations such as cupping, moxibustion, acupuncture and massage, or doing meditation and physical exercise such as *qigong*.

For example, if a woman is sick or weak from a lack of *yin qi*, she can eat foods high in *yin qi* such as melons or goji berries or various *yin*-supplementing herbs. Older men may want to take herbal and food remedies, such as drinking ginseng tea or eating seahorse dishes, because they are high in *yang* content, or get a moxibustion treatment that adds *yang* to the body.

If, due to injury or stress, the *qi* circulation gets blocked or stagnated, all the medical techniques above can be used to unblock the *qi* channels called meridians, or increase or decrease the *qi* in various locations. However, a medical practitioner should help you decide which procedure will best help to cure your condition.

Qigong and *taijiquan* practitioners think that special exercises and meditation help the *qi* in the body to circulate. They think that by practicing them people can learn to control the motion of *qi*, and use the *qi* to heal injured body parts, cure diseases, get healthier, defend themselves, and live longer.

The Most Common Techniques

Acupuncture: This strange and famous medical technique involves inserting needles into precise meridian points.

Cupping: This ancient practice isn't just a Chinese tradition, but has been practiced for hundreds and thousands of years across Eurasia and North Africa. The Chinese style uses the acupuncture meridians. It is used to remove *yang* from the body, and it is appropriate for conditions such as bronchitis, heart stroke, and conditions related to hot weather.

Herbal medicine: In many ways, Chinese herbal medicine is similar to Western herbal medicine, though the emphasis is on promoting the *yin-yang* balance.

Massage: It seems like there are massage clinics everywhere, and there are various styles that are all thought to be good for the health, some of which are more appreciated by Chinese than foreigners.

Medicinal cuisine therapy: It focuses on the traditional method of meal preparation, special recipes, and way of eating to promote the *yin-yang* balance.

Moxibustion: This is another surprising technique and is used to add *yang* to the body. It is appropriate for women with birthing problems, older men, and health issues related to cold weather. The mugwort smoke is thought to have medicinal properties.

Qigong: Meditation and special exercises, such as *Qigong* and *taijiquan*, also manipulate the *qi* balance and the body fluids in the body.

New Words

cultivation [ˌkʌltɪˈveɪʃn] *n.*	培养
sustainability [səˌsteɪnəˈbɪləti] *n.*	持续性
disharmony [dɪsˈhɑːməni] *n.*	不调和，不融洽
collapse [kəˈlæps] *v.*	使倒塌，使崩溃
holism [ˈhəʊlɪzəm] *n.*	整体论
interact [ˌɪntərˈækt] *v.*	互相影响，互相作用
optimize [ˈɒptɪmaɪz] *v.*	使最优化；使完善
descendent [dɪˈsendənt] *n.*	派生物
inception [ɪnˈsepʃn] *n.*	开端，初期
utilize [ˈjuːtəlaɪz] *v.*	利用
treatise [ˈtriːtɪs] *n.*	专著；论述
originate [əˈrɪdʒɪneɪt] *v.*	发源，发生
ascribe [əˈskraɪb] *v.*	归因于，归咎于
extraordinarily [ɪkˈstrɔːdnrəli] ad*v.*	格外地，非凡地
exhaustive [ɪgˈzɔːstɪv] *adj.*	详尽的，彻底的
moxibustion [ˌmɒksɪˈbʌstʃ(ə)n] *n.*	艾灸
massage [ˈmæsɑːʒ] *n.*	按摩
meditation [ˌmedɪˈteɪʃn] *n.*	沉思，深思
meridian [məˈrɪdiən] *n.*	经脉
bronchitis [brɒŋˈkaɪtɪs] *n.*	支气管炎
cuisine [kwɪˈziːn] *n.*	烹饪，烹调法

TEXT B   Acupuncture, Moxibustion and *Tuina*

Acupuncture, moxibustion and *tuina* are commonly used in Chinese medicine to treat diseases. Based on the theory of meridians, these methods can dredge the channels and collaterals, restore the balance between *yin* and *yang*, coordinate the functions of *zang-fu* organs, and support the healthy *qi* and eliminate the evil *qi*.

Acupuncture

Acupuncture is a therapy in which needles are inserted into certain acupoints to regulate *yin*, *yang*, *qi* and blood to treat diseases. The needles used today are often made of stainless steel which has high intensity and elasticity. Before treatment, the physician should give a full explanation to the patient in order to eliminate fear and anxiety related to acupuncture.

Selection of needles. Using proper needles is one of the most important steps to obtain a good therapeutic effect. Needles are chosen based on patient constitution, age, point location, and the condition to be treated. For example, thick long needles are selected for males or obese persons, and short thin needles are chosen for females or feeble patients.

Posture selection of the patient. Postures in the acupuncture clinic are usually divided into sitting and lying down positions. The lying down posture is further categorized into supine, lateral recumbent and prone positions. The sitting posture is subdivided into supine sitting, sitting in flexion and lateral sitting.

Methods of needle insertion. In clinical practice, physicians usually use the right hand to hold the handle of the needle with the thumb, index and middle fingers. The left hand is usually applied to press down the skin around the acupoints to support the insertion of the needles. During needle insertion, the finger force has to be gathered and passed down to the tip of the needle in order to pass the needle through the skin smoothly.

Needle manipulations. Needle manipulations refer to maneuvers conducted on a needle to promote or regulate the needling sensation, or to fulfill a reinforcing or reducing formula. They are divided into basic needle manipulations which include lifting, thrusting, twirling and rotating, and assistant manipulations such as pushing channel, scraping, flicking and shaking needle, etc.

Moxibustion

Moxibustion is a therapy which prevents and treats diseases by means of moxa wool. Moxa comes in cones or sticks. The combustion of the moxa wool permits transmission of heat to designated meridians or points of the human body for the purpose of warming the meridians and collaterals, invigorating the flow of *qi* and blood, strengthening the body resistance and eliminating evil from the body.

A moxa cone placed directly on the point and ignited is called direct moxibustion. Direct moxibustion is divided into scarring and non-scarring. In scarring moxibustion the skin is burnt and blistered, leaving a scar. In the non-scarring version, moxibustion is conducted on the points but will not cause burning, blistering and scarring. The ignited moxa cone does not contact the skin directly, but is insulated from the skin by ginger, salt, garlic, and monkshood cake.

The moxibustion process includes rolling the moxa wool with a sheet of paper into a moxa stick, applying a burning moxa stick at a certain distance apart over the selected point. There are two forms: mild-warm moxibustion and sparrow-pecking moxibustion. The former involves igniting a moxa stick at one end and placing it two to three centimeters away from the skin over the site to bring mild warmth, but not burning, for fifteen minutes until the skin becomes slightly red. Mild-warm moxibustion is suitable for all the syndromes indicated for moxibustion. In sparrow-pecking moxibustion the ignited moxa stick is moved up and down over the point like a bird pecking or moving left and right, or circularly. This form of moxibustion is indicated for numbness and pain in the limbs.

Tuina Manipulations

Tuina manipulations are a direct means of manual therapy. There are many kinds of operating skills and various forms of movements in *tuina*. Movements include butting with the head and tramping under the foot as well as continuous manipulations conducted with the finger, palm, wrist and elbow. They are directly applied to the body surface and stimulate the body by means of exerting force to prevent and treat diseases. Since most of the manipulations are done with hands, they are generally called manual manipulations or hand manipulations.

Tuina manipulations should be persistent, forceful, even and gentle. Persistence means that manipulations should be continued for a considerable period of time. Forcefulness means that manipulations should be performed with adequate force. Evenness means that manipulations should be rhythmic with appropriate speed and steady force. Gentleness refers to light but not superficial, heavy but not unsmooth operations with natural and smooth shift of movements, which should by no means be performed roughly and violently. The four points mentioned previously are organically related to one another. To skillfully command various manipulations it is necessary to carry out long and persistent exercise and practice. In practice, the exercises should be done in an orderly step by step manner, following a progression from inexperienced to skillful, to perfect and proficient.

In order to obtain better curative action in practical application, *tuina* manipulations should follow the TCM principle of differentiating syndromes to decide treatment. This requires applying different hand manipulations to different syndromes. Therapy may be differentiated based on the age of the person, old or young; weak or strong constitution; asthenia or sthenia syndromes; large or small size of the operated parts; and thick or thin muscles. Selection of manipulations and application of force should be adapted to these conditions. Any excess or deficiency in manipulation will affect the preventive and curative results or even cause some side effects.

Chinese *tuina* has a long history, dating back to the ancient times. Its manipulations date back several hundred years. Compound manipulations are formed by combining two types of manipulation with pressing and rubbing, palm twisting and kneading, or pinching and grasping. These compound manipulations are even more helpful in improving therapeutic efficacy.

New Words

collateral [kə'lætərəl] *n.*	络脉
coordinate [kəʊ'ɔːdɪneɪt] *v.*	协调，调整
acupoint ['ækjʊpɒɪnt] *n.*	穴位
elasticity [ˌiːlæ'stɪsəti] *n.*	弹性，弹力
constitution [ˌkɒnstɪ'tjuːʃn] *n.*	体格
feeble ['fiːbl] *adj.*	微弱的，虚弱的
recumbent [rɪ'kʌmbənt] *adj.*	斜倚的；休息的
ignite [ɪg'naɪt] *v.*	点火；燃烧
insulate ['ɪnsjuleɪt] *v.*	隔离，使孤立
monkshood ['mʌŋkshʊd] *n.*	舟形乌头
butt [bʌt] *v.*	以头抵撞
tramp [træmp] *v.*	践踏，踩
differentiate [ˌdɪfə'renʃieɪt] *v.*	区分，区别
asthenia [əs'θiːnɪə] *n.*	无力，衰弱
sthenia [sθɪ'naɪə] *n.*	强壮

FOLLOW–UP ACTIVITIES

Translation

A.Translate the following sentences into Chinese.

1. Thus TCM not only identifies and treats illness and prevents disease but, just as importantly, optimizes health, well-being, and sustainability in our lives and in our world.

_____

_____

2. In many ways, Chinese herbal medicine is similar to Western herbal medicine, though the emphasis is on promoting the *yin-yang* balance.

_____

_____

3. Before treatment, the physician should give a full explanation to the patient in order to eliminate fear and anxiety related to acupuncture.

_____

_____

4. They are directly applied to the body surface and stimulate the body by means of exerting force to prevent and treat diseases.

_____

_____

B. Translate the following sentences into English.

1. 阴阳消长，是指相互对立、相互依存的阴阳双方不是静止不变的，而是处于动态变化之中。

_____

_____

2. 阳盛则热，阴盛则寒；阳虚生外寒，阴虚生内热。

_____

_____

3. 问诊是中医诊断中的一个重要手段，可以为确定疾病的阴阳、表里、寒热及虚实提供重要依据。

_____

_____

4. 拔罐被广泛用于治疗感冒、呼吸道感染、哮喘、腹泻以及其他内脏疾病，具有缓解肌肉痉挛、刺激血液循环，以及提高免疫力的功能。

_____

_____

NCLEX–RN® Test Format

The only way to work as a licensed registered nurse is by passing the National Council Licensure Examination (NCLEX-RN® exam). In other words, if you don't pass the NCLEX-RN® exam, you can't work as an RN.

The NCLEX-RN® has one purpose: To determine if it's safe for you to begin practice as an entry-level nurse. It is significantly different from any test that you took in nursing school. While nursing school exams are knowledge-based, the NCLEX-RN® tests application and analysis using the nursing knowledge you learned in school. You will be tested on how you can use critical thinking skills to make nursing judgments.

Framework

The NCLEX-RN® exam is organized according to the framework, "Meeting Client Needs". There are four major categories and eight subcategories. Many nursing programs are based on the medical model where students take separate medical, surgical, pediatric, psychiatric, and obstetric classes. However, on the NCLEX-RN® exam, all of the content is integrated.

Types of Questions

Questions are primarily multiple-choice with four possible answer choices; however, there are also alternate question types. Alternate question types include but are not limited to multiple-response, fill-in-the-blank, calculation, ordered response, and/or hot spots. All question types may include multimedia such as charts, tables, graphics, sound and video. All questions go through an extensive review process before being used as questions on the examination.

Taking the NCLEX-RN® Exam

How many questions are there?

All registered nurse candidates must answer a minimum of 75 questions. The maximum number of questions that a registered nurse candidate may answer is 265 during the allotted six-hour time period. The maximum six-hour time limit to complete the examination includes the tutorial, sample questions and all breaks. Regardless of how many you answer, you will be given 15 experimental questions that do not count for or against you. The exam administrators use them to test for future questions on the exam.

How much time will I have?

There is no time limit for each individual question. You'll have a maximum of 6 hours to complete the exam, which includes the tutorial, sample questions and all breaks. There are no mandatory breaks. However, there's an optional break after 2.5 hours of testing, and another optional break after 3.5 hours of testing.

When does the exam end?

Your exam ends when one of the following occurs:

● You have demonstrated minimum competency and answered the minimum number of questions (75).

● You have demonstrated a lack of minimum competency and answered the minimum number of questions (75).

● You have answered the maximum number of questions (265).

● You have used the maximum time allowed (6 hours).

TIP: Try not to focus on the length of your exam. You should just plan on testing for 6 hours and completing 265 questions. And if you have a long exam, remember that you are still in the game as long as the computer continues to give you questions; so focus on answering them all to the best of your ability.

Taking the NCLEX-RN® CAT

The NCLEX-RN® Examination is administered to candidates by computerized adaptive testing (CAT). CAT is a method of delivering examinations that uses computer technology and measurement theory. With CAT, each candidate's examination is unique because it is assembled interactively as the examination proceeds. Computer technology selects items to administer that match the candidate's ability. The questions, which are stored in a large item pool, have been classified by test plan category and level of difficulty. After the candidate answers the question, the computer calculates an ability estimate based on all of the previous answers the candidate selected. The next question administered is chosen to measure the candidate's ability in the appropriate test plan category. This process is repeated for each question, creating an examination tailored to the candidate's knowledge and skills while fulfilling all NCLEX-RN® Test Plan requirements. The examination continues with items selected and administered in this way until a pass or fail decision is made. In other words, based on your skill level, the CAT ensures that the questions are not "too hard" or "too easy". Your first question will be relatively easy--below the level of minimum competency. If you answer it correctly, the computer selects a slightly more difficult question. If answered incorrectly, the computer selects a slightly easier question. By continuing to do this throughout the test, the computer is able to determine your level of competence.

NCLEX-RN® Grading System

Pass/Fail

The NCLEX-RN® exam is pass/fail—there is no numerical score. A determination will be made at the conclusion of the exam as to whether you have passed or failed. However, the results will not be made available at the exam site. You'll be notified by your State Board of Nursing approximately 4-6 weeks after your test date.

What if I fail?

First, don't despair. You are not alone. Many students do not pass the NCLEX-RN® exam on their first attempt. Failing the exam means that you did not successfully answer questions at or above the level of difficulty needed to pass. On this particular exam, you were unable to demonstrate your ability to provide safe and effective care.

If you fail, you'll receive a diagnostic profile that evaluates your test performance. Read it carefully. You'll see how many questions you answered on the exam. The more questions you answered, the closer you came to passing.

The only way you continue to get questions after the first 75 is if you are answering questions close to the level of difficulty need to pass. Use the diagnostic profile to determine your problem areas. You can then focus your preparation accordingly.

Should I test again?

Absolutely. Re-testing for the NCLEX-RN® exam is permitted 45 days after the initial administration (unless you're in Georgia or Guam—contact SBON for details).

If you prepared on your own for the first time, you may want to consider a formal preparation option to help you focus your study time more effectively.

Regardless of the method you choose, don't forget to use the diagnostic profile to guide your preparation.

How to Register for the NCLEX-RN®

1. Submit an application for licensure/registration to the board of nursing (BON) where you wish to be licensed/registered.

2. Meet all of the BON's eligibility requirements to take the NCLEX.

3. Register for the NCLEX with Pearson VUE.

4. Receive NCLEX Registration Acknowledgement email from Pearson VUE.

5. The BON makes you eligible in the Pearson VUE system.

6. Receive Authorization to Test (ATT) email from Pearson VUE.

7. Schedule your exam with Pearson VUE.

Please note that all correspondence from Pearson VUE will arrive only by email.

NCLEX–RN® Exam Structure

Distribution of Content for the NCLEX–RN® Exam

Client Needs	Percentage of Items from Each Category/Subcategory
Safe and Effective Care Environment	
• Management of Care	17% ~ 23%
• Safety and Infection Control	9% ~ 15%
Health Promotion and Maintenance	6% ~ 12%
Psychosocial Integrity	6% ~ 12%

Client Needs	Percentage of Items from Each Category/Subcategory
Physiological Integrity	
● Basic Care and Comfort	6% ～ 12%
● Pharmacological and Parenteral Therapies	12% ～ 18%
● Reduction of Risk Potential	9% ～ 15%
● Physiological Adaptation	11% ～ 17%

Overview of Content

All content categories and subcategories reflect client needs across the life span in a variety of settings.

Safe and Effective Care Environment

The nurse promotes achievement of client outcomes by providing and directing nursing care that enhances the care delivery setting in order to protect clients and health care personnel.

● Management of Care—providing and directing nursing care that enhances the care delivery setting to protect clients and health care personnel.

Related content includes but is **not limited** to:

● Advance Directives/Self-Determination/Life Planning.

● Assignment, Delegation and Supervision.

● Establishing Priorities.

● Advocacy.

● Ethical Practice.

● Case Management.

● Informed Consent.

● Client Rights.

● Information Technology.

● Organ Donation.

● Collaboration with Interdisciplinary Team.

● Legal Rights and Responsibilities.

● Confidentiality/Information Security.

● Concepts of Management.

● Continuity of Care.

● Performance Improvement (Quality Improvement).

● Referrals.

● Safety and Infection Control—protecting clients and health care personnel from health and environmental hazards.

Related content includes but is **not limited** to:

● Accident/Error/Injury Prevention.

- Emergency Response Plan
- Safe Use of Equipment.
- Security Plan.
- Ergonomic Principles.
- Home Safety.
- Standard Precautions/Transmission-Based Precautions/Surgical Asepsis.
- Handling Hazardous and Infectious Materials.
- Reporting of Incident/Event/Irregular Occurrence/Variance.
- Use of Restraints/Safety Devices.

Health Promotion and Maintenance

The nurse provides and directs nursing care of the client that incorporates the knowledge of expected growth and development principles; prevention and/or early detection of health problems, and strategies to achieve optimal health.

Related content includes but is **not limited** to:

- Aging Process.
- High Risk Behaviors.
- Ante/Intra/Postpartum and Newborn Care.
- Lifestyle Choices.
- Developmental Stages and Transitions.
- Self-Care.
- Health Promotion/Disease Prevention.
- Health Screening.
- Techniques of Physical Assessment.

Psychosocial Integrity

The nurse provides and directs nursing care that promotes and supports the emotional, mental and social wellbeing of the client experiencing stressful events, as well as clients with acute or chronic mental illness.

Related content includes but is **not limited** to:

- Abuse/Neglect.
- Family Dynamics.
- Behavioral Interventions.
- Grief and Loss.
- Chemical and Other Dependencies/ Substance Use Disorder.
- Religious and Spiritual Influences on Health.
- Coping Mechanisms.
- Sensory/Perceptual Alterations.
- Crisis Intervention.
- Stress Management.
- Mental Health Concepts.
- Therapeutic Communication.

- Therapeutic Environment.
- End of Life Care.
- Support Systems.
- Cultural Awareness/Cultural Influences on Health.

Physiological Integrity

The nurse promotes physical health and wellness by providing care and comfort, reducing client risk potential and managing health alterations.

● Basic Care and Comfort— providing comfort and assistance in the performance of activities of daily living.

Related content includes but is **not limited** to:

- Assistive Devices.
- Nutrition and Oral Hydration.
- Elimination.
- Personal Hygiene.
- Mobility/Immobility.
- Rest and Sleep.
- Non-Pharmacological Comfort Interventions.

● Pharmacological and Parenteral Therapies - providing care related to the administration of medications and parenteral therapies.

Related content includes but is **not limited** to:

- Adverse Effects/Contraindications/Side Effects/Interactions.
- Expected Actions/Outcomes.
- Medication Administration.
- Blood and Blood Products.
- Parenteral/Intravenous Therapies.
- Central Venous Access Devices.
- Pharmacological Pain Management.
- Dosage Calculation.
- Total Parenteral Nutrition.

● Reduction of Risk Potential—reducing the likelihood that clients will develop complications or health problems related to existing conditions, treatments or procedures.

Related content includes but is **not limited** to:

- Changes/Abnormalities in Vital Signs.
- Diagnostic Tests.
- Potential for Complications from Surgical Procedures and Health Alterations.
- Laboratory Values.
- System Specific Assessments.
- Potential for Alterations in Body Systems.
- Therapeutic Procedures.
- Potential for Complications of Diagnostic Tests/Treatments/Procedures.

● Physiological Adaptation—managing and providing care for clients with acute, chronic or life threatening physical health conditions.

Related content includes but is **not limited** to:

- Alterations in Body Systems.
- Medical Emergencies.
- Fluid and Electrolyte Imbalances.
- Pathophysiology.
- Hemodynamics.
- Unexpected Response to Therapies.

NCLEX–RN® Practice Questions Set 1

1. A patient arrives at the emergency department complaining of mid-sternal chest pain. Which of the following nursing actions should take priority?

A. A complete history with emphasis on preceding events.

B. An electrocardiogram.

C. Careful assessment of vital signs.

D. Chest exam with auscultation.

2. A patient has been hospitalized with pneumonia and is about to be discharged. A nurse provides discharge instructions to a patient and his family. Which misunderstanding by the family indicates the need for more detailed information?

A. The patient may resume normal home activities as tolerated but should avoid physical exertion and get adequate rest.

B. The patient should resume a normal diet with emphasis on nutritious, healthy foods.

C. The patient may discontinue the prescribed course of oral antibiotics once the symptoms have completely resolved.

D. The patient should continue use of the incentive spirometer to keep airways open and free of secretions.

3. A nurse is caring for an elderly Vietnamese patient in the terminal stages of lung cancer. Many family members are in the room around the clock performing unusual rituals and bringing ethnic foods. Which of the following actions should the nurse take?

A. Restrict visiting hours and ask the family to limit visitors to two at a time.

B. Notify visitors with a sign on the door that the patient is limited to clear fluids only with no solid food allowed.

C. If possible, keep the other bed in the room unassigned to provide privacy and comfort to the family.

D. Contact the physician to report the unusual rituals and activities.

4. The charge nurse on the cardiac unit is planning assignments for the day. Which of the following is the most appropriate assignment for the float nurse that has been reassigned from labor and delivery?

A. A one-week postoperative coronary bypass patient, who is being evaluated for placement of a pacemaker prior to discharge.

B. A suspected myocardial infarction patient on telemetry, just admitted from the Emergency Department and scheduled for an angiogram.

C. A patient with unstable angina being closely monitored for pain and medication titration.

D. A post-operative valve replacement patient who was recently admitted to the unit because all surgical beds were filled.

5. A newly diagnosed 8-year-old child with type I diabetes mellitus and his mother are receiving diabetes education prior to discharge. The physician has prescribed Glucagon for emergency use. The mother asks the purpose of this medication. Which of the following statements by the nurse is correct?

A. Glucagon enhances the effect of insulin in case the blood sugar remains high one hour after injection.

B. Glucagon treats hypoglycemia resulting from insulin overdose.

C. Glucagon treats lipoatrophy from insulin injections.

D. Glucagon prolongs the effect of insulin, allowing fewer injections.

6. A patient on the cardiac telemetry unit unexpectedly goes into ventricular fibrillation. The advanced cardiac life support team prepares to defibrillate. Which of the following choices indicates the correct placement of the conductive gel pads?

A. The left clavicle and right lower sternum.

B. Right of midline below the bottom rib and the left shoulder.

C. The upper and lower halves of the sternum.

D. The right side of the sternum just below the clavicle and left of the precordium.

7. The nurse performs an initial abdominal assessment on a patient newly admitted for abdominal pain. The nurse hears what she describes as "clicks and gurgles in all four quadrants" as well as "swishing or buzzing sound heard in one or two quadrants." Which of the following statements is correct?

A. The frequency and intensity of bowel sounds varies depending on the phase of digestion.

B. In the presence of intestinal obstruction, bowel sounds will be louder and higher pitched.

C. A swishing or buzzing sound may represent the turbulent blood flow of a bruit and is not normal.

D. All of the above.

8. A patient arrives in the emergency department and reports splashing concentrated household cleaner in his eye. Which of the following nursing actions is a priority?

A. Irrigate the eye repeatedly with normal saline solution.

B. Place fluorescein drops in the eye.

C. Patch the eye.

D. Test visual acuity.

9. A nurse is caring for a patient who has had hip replacement. The nurse should be most concerned about which of the following findings?

A. Complaints of pain during repositioning.

B. Scant bloody discharge on the surgical dressing.

C. Complaints of pain following physical therapy.

D. Temperature of 101.8 °F (38.7℃).

10. A child is admitted to the hospital with an uncontrolled seizure disorder. The admitting physician writes orders for actions to be taken in the event of a seizure. Which of the following actions would NOT be included?

A. Notify the physician.

B. Restrain the patient's limbs.

C. Position the patient on his/her side with the head flexed forward.

D. Administer rectal diazepam.

11. Emergency department triage is an important nursing function. A nurse working the evening shift is presented with four patients at the same time. Which of the following patients should be assigned the highest priority?

A. A patient with low-grade fever, headache, and myalgias for the past 72 hours.

B. A patient who is unable to bear weight on the left foot, with swelling and bruising following a running accident.

C. A patient with abdominal and chest pain following a large, spicy meal.

D. A child with a one-inch bleeding laceration on the chin but otherwise well after falling while jumping on his bed.

12. A patient is admitted to the hospital with a calcium level of 6.0 mg/dL. Which of the following symptoms would you NOT expect to see in this patient?

A. Numbness in hands and feet.

B. Muscle cramping.

C. Hypoactive bowel sounds.

D. Positive Chvostek's sign.

13. A nurse cares for a patient who has a nasogastric tube attached to low suction because of a suspected bowel obstruction. Which of the following arterial blood gas results might be expected in this patient?

A. pH 7.52, PCO2 54 mm Hg.

B. pH 7.42, PCO2 40 mm Hg.

C. pH 7.25, PCO2 25 mm Hg.

D. pH 7.38, PCO2 36 mm Hg.

14. A patient is admitted to the hospital for routine elective surgery. Included in the list of current medications is Coumadin (warfarin) at a high dose. Concerned about the possible effects of the drug, particularly in a patient scheduled for surgery, the nurse anticipates which of the following actions?

A. Draw a blood sample for prothrombin (PT) and international normalized ratio (INR) level.

B. Administer vitamin K.

C. Draw a blood sample for type and crossmatch and request blood from the blood bank.

D. Cancel the surgery after the patient reports stopping the Coumadin one week previously.

15. The following lab results are received for a patient. Which of the following results are abnormal? Note: More than one answer may be correct.

A. Hemoglobin 10.4 g/dL.

B. Total cholesterol 340 mg/dL.

C. Total serum protein 7.0 g/dL.

D. Glycosylated hemoglobin A1C 5.4%.

16. A nurse is performing routine assessment of an IV site in a patient receiving both IV fluids and medications through the line. Which of the following would indicate the need for discontinuation of the IV line as the next nursing action?

A. The patient complains of pain on movement.

B. The area proximal to the insertion site is reddened, warm, and painful.

C. The IV solution is infusing too slowly, particularly when the limb is elevated.

D. A hematoma is visible in the area of the IV insertion site.

17. A hospitalized patient has received transfusions of 2 units of blood over the past few hours. A nurse enters the room to find the patient sitting up in bed, dyspneic and uncomfortable. On assessment, crackles are heard in the bases of both lungs, probably indicating that the patient is experiencing a complication of transfusion. Which of the following complications is most likely the cause of the patient's symptoms?

A. Febrile non-hemolytic reaction.

B. Allergic transfusion reaction.

C. Acute hemolytic reaction.

D. Fluid overload.

18. A patient in labor and delivery has just received an amniotomy. Which of the following is correct? Note: More than one answer may be correct.

A. Frequent checks for cervical dilation will be needed after the procedure.

B. Contractions may rapidly become stronger and closer together after the procedure.

C. The FHR (fetal heart rate) will be followed closely after the procedure due to the possibility of cord compression.

D. The procedure is usually painless and is followed by a gush of amniotic fluid.

19. A nurse is counseling the mother of a newborn infant with hyperbilirubinemia. Which of the following instructions by the nurse is NOT correct?

A. Continue to breastfeed frequently, at least every 2-4 hours.

B. Follow up with the infant's physician within 72 hours of discharge for a recheck of the serum bilirubin and exam.

C. Watch for signs of dehydration, including decreased urinary output and changes in skin turgor.

D. Keep the baby quiet and swaddled, and place the bassinet in a dimly lit area.

20. A nurse is giving discharge instructions to the parents of a healthy newborn. Which of the following instructions should the nurse provide regarding car safety and the trip home from the hospital?

A. The infant should be restrained in an infant car seat, properly secured in the back seat in a rear-facing position.

B. The infant should be restrained in an infant car seat, properly secured in the front passenger seat.

C. The infant should be restrained in an infant car seat facing forward or rearward in the back seat.

D. For the trip home from the hospital, the parent may sit in the back seat and hold the newborn.

NCLEX–RN® Practice Questions Set 2

1. A mother complains to the clinic nurse that her 2 ½-year-old son is not yet toilet trained. She is particularly concerned that, although he reliably uses the potty seat for bowel movements, he isn't able to hold his urine for long periods. Which of the following statements by the nurse is correct?

A. The child should have been trained by age 2 and may have a psychological problem that is responsible for his "accidents."

B. Bladder control is usually achieved before bowel control, and the child should be required to sit on the potty seat until he passes urine.

C. Bowel control is usually achieved before bladder control, and the average age for completion of toilet training varies widely from 24 to 36 months.

D. The child should be told "no" each time he wets so that he learns the behavior is unacceptable.

2. The mother of a 14-month-old child reports to the nurse that her child will not fall asleep at night without a bottle of milk in the crib and often wakes during the night asking for another. Which of the following instructions by the nurse is correct?

A. Allow the child to have the bottle at bedtime, but withhold the one later in the night.

B. Put juice in the bottle instead of milk.

C. Give only a bottle of water at bedtime.

D. Do not allow bottles in the crib.

3. Which of the following actions is NOT appropriate in the care of a 2-month-old infant?

A. Place the infant on her back for naps and bedtime.

B. Allow the infant to cry for 5 minutes before responding if she wakes during the night as she may fall back asleep.

C. Talk to the infant frequently and make eye contact to encourage language development.

D. Wait until at least 4 months to add infant cereals and strained fruits to the diet.

4. An older patient asks a nurse to recommend strategies to prevent constipation. Which of the following suggestions would be helpful? Note: More than one answer may be correct.

A. Get moderate exercise for at least 30 minutes each day.

B. Drink 6-8 glasses of water each day.

C. Eat a diet high in fiber.

D. Take a mild laxative if you don't have a bowel movement every day.

5. A child is admitted to the hospital with suspected rheumatic fever. Which of the following observations is NOT the confirmation of the diagnosis?

A. A reddened rash visible over the trunk and extremities.

B. A history of sore throat that was self-limited in the past month.

C. A negative antistreptolysin O titer.

D. An unexplained fever.

6. An infant with congestive heart failure is receiving diuretic therapy at home. Which of the following symptoms would indicate that the dosage may need to be increased?

A. Sudden weight gain.

B. Decreased blood pressure.

C. Slow, shallow breathing.

D. Bradycardia.

7. A patient taking Dilantin (phenytoin) for a seizure disorder is experiencing breakthrough seizures. A blood sample is taken to determine the serum drug level. Which of the following would indicate a sub-therapeutic level?

A. 15 mcg/mL.

B. 4 mcg/mL.

C. 10 mcg/dL.

D. 5 mcg/dL.

8. A patient arrives at the emergency department complaining of back pain. He reports taking at least 3 acetaminophen tablets every three hours for the past week without relief. Which of the following symptoms suggests acetaminophen toxicity?

A. Tinnitus.

B. Diarrhea.

C. Hypertension.

D. Hepatic damage.

9. A nurse is caring for a cancer patient receiving subcutaneous morphine sulfate for pain. Which of the following nursing actions is the most important in the care of this patient?

A. Monitor urine output.

B. Monitor respiratory rate.

C. Monitor heart rate.

D. Monitor temperature.

10. A patient arrives at the emergency department with severe lower leg pain after a fall in a touch football game. Following routine triage, which of the following is the appropriate next step in assessment and treatment?

A. Apply heat to the painful area.

B. Apply an elastic bandage to the leg.

C. X-ray the leg.

D. Give pain medication.

11. A nurse is evaluating a post-operative patient and notes a moderate amount of serous drainage on the dressing 24 hours after surgery. Which of the following is the appropriate nursing action?

A. Notify the surgeon about evidence of infection immediately.

B. Leave the dressing intact to avoid disturbing the wound site.

C. Remove the dressing and leave the wound site open to air.

D. Change the dressing and document the clean appearance of the wound site.

12. A patient returns to the emergency department less than 24 hours after having a fiberglass cast applied for a fractured right radius. Which of the following patient complaints would cause the nurse to be concerned about impaired perfusion to the limb?

A. Severe itching under the cast.

B. Severe pain in the right shoulder.

C. Severe pain in the right lower arm.

D. Increased warmth in the fingers.

13. An older patient with osteoarthritis is preparing for discharge. Which of the following information is correct.

A. Increased physical activity and daily exercise will help decrease discomfort associated with the condition.

B. Joint pain will diminish after a full night of rest.

C. Nonsteroidal anti-inflammatory medications should be taken on an empty stomach.

D. Acetaminophen (Tylenol) is a more effective anti-inflammatory than ibuprofen (Motrin).

14. Which patient should NOT be prescribed alendronate (Fosamax) for osteoporosis?

A. A female patient being treated for high blood pressure with an ACE inhibitor.

B. A patient who is allergic to iodine/shellfish.

C. A patient on a calorie restricted diet.

D. A patient on bed rest who must maintain a supine position.

15. Which of the following strategies is NOT effective for prevention of Lyme disease?

A. Insect repellant on the skin and clothes when in a Lyme endemic area.

B. Long sleeved shirts and long pants.

C. Prophylactic antibiotic therapy prior to anticipated exposure to ticks.

D. Careful examination of skin and hair for ticks following anticipated exposure.

16. A nurse is counseling patients at a health clinic on the importance of immunizations. Which of the following information is the most accurate regarding immunizations?

A. All infectious diseases can be prevented with proper immunization.

B. Immunizations provide natural immunity from disease.

C. Immunizations are risk-free and should be universally administered.

D. Immunization provides acquired immunity from some specific diseases.

17. A patient is brought to the emergency department after a bee sting. The family reports a history of severe allergic reaction, and the patient appears to have some oral swelling. Which of the following is the most urgent nursing action?

A. Consult a physician.

B. Maintain a patent airway.

C. Administer epinephrine subcutaneously.

D. Administer diphenhydramine (Benadryl) orally.

18. A mother calls the clinic to report that her son has recently started medication to treat

attention deficit/hyperactivity disorder (ADHD). The mother fears her son is experiencing side effects of the medicine. Which of the following side effects are typically related to medications used for ADHD? Note: More than one answer may be correct:

A. Poor appetite.

B. Insomnia.

C. Sleepiness.

D. Agitation.

19. A patient at a mental health clinic is taking Haldol (haloperidol) for treatment of schizophrenia. She calls the clinic to report abnormal movements of her face and tongue. Which of the following symptoms cloes the nurse conclude that the patient is experiencing?

A. Co-morbid depression.

B. Psychotic hallucinations.

C. Negative symptoms of schizophrenia.

D. Tardive dyskinesia.

20. A patient with newly diagnosed diabetes mellitus is learning to recognize the symptoms of hypoglycemia. Which of the following symptoms is indicative of hypoglycemia?

A. Polydipsia.

B. Confusion.

C. Blurred vision.

D. Polyphagia.

What You Need to Know About NCLEX

The facts about NCLEX that you should know.

Purpose

● *To determine if you are a safe and effective nurse.*

● *To safeguard the public.*

● *To test for minimum competency.*

Test Content

● *Based on the knowledge and activities of an entry-level nurse.*

● *Written by nursing faculty and clinical specialists.*

● *Presented as multiple-choice questions with four possible answer choices.*

● *Based on integrated nursing content – not on the medical model of medical, surgical, obstetrics, pediatrics, and psychiatric nursing.*

● *Includes 15 experimental questions.*

Test Administration

● *The computer adaptive test adapts to your knowledge, skills, and ability level.*

● *The question sequence is determined interactively.*

● *Questions are selected based on the item difficulty and the test plan.*

● *Test dates and times are individually scheduled through a Sylvan Learning Center.*

● *Tests are administered at individual computer stations.*

Taking the Exam

● *Computer knowledge is not required.*

● *2 keys are used: the space bar to move the cursor and enter/return to highlight and lock in your answer.*

● *All other computer keys are disconnected.*

● *You receive instructions and a practice exercise before beginning the exam.*

● *Any necessary background information appears on the screen with the question.*

● *The computer selects a relatively easy first question.*

● *The next question is selected by the computer based on your response to the first question.*

● *If your answer is correct, the next question is slightly more difficult.*

● *If your answer is incorrect, the next question is slightly easier.*

● *Questions are selected to precisely measure your ability in each area of the test plan.*

Timing

● *There is no time limit for each individual question.*

● *You will answer a minimum of 75 questions to a maximum of 265 questions.*

● *The maximum time for the exam is 6 hours, including the practice exercise and all breaks.*

This Exam Will End

● *When the computer has determined your ability, or*

● *When a maximum of 6 hours of testing is reached, or*

● *When a maximum of 265 questions have been answered.*

Scoring

● *It is a pass/fail exam.*

● *There is no penalty for guessing.*

● *The 15 experimental questions are not counted.*

Concerns

● *No answer changes. Questions are selected by the computer based on your previous responses.*

● *No scrolling back.*

● *No skipping questions. You must answer the question to go on.*

Advantages

● *Testing is available year-round, 15 hours a day, six days a week, in six-hour time slots.*

● *Results are released by individual state boards.*

● *If you fail, you can retest 45 days after the initial testing.*

Appendix 1
Keys to Exercises

Unit One

A. Translate the following sentences into Chinese.

1. 护理涵盖了促进健康，预防疾病，以及对疾病患者、伤残患者和临终患者所提供的护理。

2. 护理不仅是一种技能，还是一个集灵魂、思想和想象力为一体的过程。

3. 总的来说，护理学反映了人类与健康和疾病的关系，涉及生物、行为、社会和文化等领域。

4. 护士的独特作用在于帮助个体（不论是患者还是健康人）进行有益于保持或恢复健康的活动（或者安详地死去），最终使这个人有足够的力量、意志和知识，可以独立完成这些活动。

B. Translate the following sentences into English.

1. Person-centered care focuses on the care of the whole person, that is, the care of body, mind, and spirit.

2. Self-awareness and self-care are core practices that are foundational to integrative nursing.

3. Helping patients is the nurse's duty. Deep inside your heart there will be a desire and drive to do something that will improve the life quality of others.

4. Nursing theory is the systematic abstraction about nursing practice, which purpose is to describe, explain, predict, and control nursing action to achieve certain nursing practice outcomes.

Unit Two

A. Translate the following sentences into Chinese.

1. 每家医院提供的服务和包括的科室各不相同。不过，医院大都包括两个主要部门：门诊部和住院部。

2. 门诊患者是指不需要住院超过 24 小时，但出于诊断或治疗目的到医院、诊所或相关机构就医的患者。这种情况下医院提供的治疗方式为非住院治疗。

3. 入院需要撰写住院记录。离开医院的正式说法为出院，需要相应的出院记录。

4. 急性间质性肾炎最常见的诱因仍然是药物，但需要谨慎地进行鉴别诊断，以便区别于其他病种。

B. Translate the following sentences into English.

1. Health care practitioners include physicians, surgeons, dentists, nurses, pharmacists, dietitians, therapists, psychologists, clinical officers, emergency medical technicians, medical laboratory scientists,

and radiographers, etc.

2. A hospital has many sections or parts, including a registration office, a dispensary (pharmacy), clinical laboratory, blood bank, central supply room, operating rooms, and radiology (X-ray and computerized tomography) rooms.

3. Avoiding medications that lead to acute interstitial nephritis may relieve symptoms quickly. Limiting salt and fluid in the diet can improve edema and high blood pressure.

4. Acute interstitial nephritis may be more severe and more likely to lead to long-term or permanent kidney damage in elderly people.

Unit Three

A. Translate the following sentences into Chinese.

1. 现病史或疾病史是最重要的因素，有助于医务人员做出诊断或确定患者的需求。

2. 呼吸困难可能是焦虑的正常表现，但也提示可能存在潜在的心肺疾病、神经肌肉疾病或过敏反应。

3. 浅部触诊法是评估表面特征的最佳方法。浅部触诊时，用指尖和指腹轻轻按压身体某一部位，然后在该部位轻轻揉动，按压的深度大约半英寸。

4. 如果你观察到患者呼吸窘迫的体征，如气短，神志不清或焦虑，应该推迟对病史的详细询问，而专注于目前紧急的问题。

5. 全身系统评估用于获取全身各个系统的现病史和既往史，可以识别患者之前未提及的健康问题。

B. Translate the following sentences into English.

1. Young children are more susceptible to respiratory infections because their airways are smaller and an unpracticed immune system, but as people age, their forced expiratory volume decreases.

2. Hypoxia, increased energy expended for breathing, and associated cardiac involvement accompany long-standing lung disease and contribute to the development of fatigue.

3. Among general observations that should be noted in the initial examination of the patient are posture and stature, body movements, nutritional status, speech pattern, and vital signs.

4. The nurse should observe the patient's face during palpation to see if palpation of any areas causes discomfort as this may be important in diagnosing a patient problem.

Unit Four

A. Translate the following sentences into Chinese.

1. 生命体征包括体温、脉率、脉律、呼吸和血压等。

2. 体温可以使用体温计进行测量。它反映了人体产热和散热之间的动态平衡。

3. 很多因素可以影响体温，如昼夜节律、压力、运动、环境温度、年龄和激素等。

4. 下面是一些与呼吸有关的术语：平静呼吸、呼吸过慢、呼吸急促、呼吸暂停、呼吸音、分泌物和咳嗽。

B. Translate the following sentences into English.

1. The pulse rate is usually taken from the radial artery at the wrist and recorded as beats per minute or measured by listening directly to the heartbeat with a stethoscope. The pulse varies with age. An

adult's pulse rate is usually between 60 and 100 beats per minute. And a newborn can have a pulse rate of about 130-150 beats per minute.

2. Vital signs are measures of various physiological conditions in order to assess the basic body functions. Abnormal vital signs may indicate a change in health. Vital signs often vary by age.

3. Blood pressure is defined as the force of the blood against arterial walls. It consists of systolic pressure and diastolic pressure. The former means the maximum blood pressure exerted on the arterial walls when the left ventricles of the heart push blood through the aortic valve into the arteries during contraction.

4. Respiratory rate is the number of breaths in one minute when the patient is at rest. To do this, count the times the chest rises for one full minute while the patient is breathing normally. The normal rate of adults is 12 to 18 breaths per minute.

Unit Five

A. Translate the following sentences into Chinese.

1. 由于癌细胞会生长到或破坏肿瘤附近的组织，压迫患者体内的骨骼、神经或其他器官，因此癌症会导致疼痛。

2. 神经阻滞是将局部麻醉剂注射到神经或其周围，可以防止疼痛信号沿着神经通路传导至大脑。

3. 有了当今癌痛的知识和各种止痛方法，人们不再遭受无法缓解的疼痛带来的痛苦。

4. 许多医生和其他医务人员可能会更关注对疾病的控制而不是对疼痛的控制。在探视患者时，他们可能不会专门询问疼痛情况，而这本该成为他们探视患者时常规询问的内容。

B. Translate the following sentences into English.

1. For acute pain, standard pain assessment scales work fairly well, but for patients with chronic pain, numeric scales are more difficult to use. A better way for nurses to gauge improvement is to ask patients with chronic pain what level of pain they experience on a daily basis. For these patients, success with pain management may need to be measured by the increase in a patient's functionality, rather than by the decrease in pain intensity.

2. The comprehensive evaluation of a patient's pain includes, but is not limited to: location, intensity, duration of the pain; aggravating and relieving factors; effects on activities of daily living, sleep pattern and psychological aspects of the patient's life; and effectiveness of current management strategies.

Unit Six

A. Translate the following sentences into Chinese.

1. 在给药时，护士务必核对患者的姓名，以便给患者使用正确的药物。

2. 根据医疗机构的政策，投药医嘱可以是手写体或计算机医嘱录入系统的打印版。

3. 为患者进行肌肉注射时，按医嘱要求准备是十分重要的。

4. 医生通常会对给药时间作出特定说明，因此护士应该在正确的时间给药。

B. Translate the following sentences into English.

1. Three checks refer to the checks before, during and after drug preparation.

2. Seven checks refer to the checks of patient's name, bed number, drug name, dose, method, concentration, and time.

3. Three checks and seven checks are the fundamental principles that nurses must uphold when administering drugs.

4. To ensure patient safety, measures must be taken to administer medications properly and to minimize medication errors.

Unit Seven

A. Translate the following sentences into Chinese.

1. 如果怀疑链球菌感染，应立即进行检测，这样才能及时给予抗感染治疗。

2. 虽然大量的数据证明了暴露后预防性给药的有效性，但仍然存在一些预防失败的案例。一般来说，失败的主要原因在于治疗延迟、暴露水平、治疗的持续时间等。

3. 例如，大便隐血试验可以检测粪便中的微量血液，有助于诊断消化道炎症、消化道出血、上消化道溃疡及结肠癌等。

4. 在排除 HIV 感染之前，你应该避免在发生性行为时出现体液接触，推迟妊娠，不要献血或捐献器官。

B. Translate the following sentences into English.

1. Based on the symptoms you have described, you need to complete a series of tests including blood routine test, urine routine test, and stool routine test.

2. When collecting throat swab specimen, burn the tube opening to sterilize it with the alcohol lamp, and then insert the long swab into the tube and stuff it up. If disinfection is not strict, it will pollute the specimen and affect the test results.

3. After the specimens are collected, they should be submitted for inspection as soon as possible to refrain from pollution.

4. Testing of blood glucose can be done by capillary blood sampling or venous blood sampling.

Unit Eight

A. Translate the following sentences into Chinese.

1. 焦虑会引起生理反应，导致血压升高、心动过速及体温升高。

2. 控制疼痛非常重要。在手术即将结束时，医生可以在手术部位注射长效止痛药，能在术后 6 ~ 12 小时内减轻疼痛。

3. 对术后预期的教育是改善患者康复结果的最好方式之一。对预期结果的宣教也可以增加依从性，有助于预防并发症。宣教内容包括让患者寻找机会练习咳嗽和深呼吸，注意固定切口。另外，应该告知患者术后早期下床活动的重要性。

4. 巡回护士给患者提供术前护理，包括术前用药、建立静脉通道、执行术前操作，如备皮和全面了解患者病史。

B. Translate the following sentences into English.

1. Bowel clearance may be ordered if the patient is having surgery of the lower gastrointestinal tract. Bowel preparation should be done early the evening before surgery to prevent interrupted sleep during the night.

2. Many factors contribute to anxiety in patients about undergoing surgery, such as the anaesthetic, the procedure itself and the potential outcome of the surgery.

3. Instruction about the surgery itself includes informing the patient about what will be done during the surgery, and how long the procedure is expected to take. The patient should be told where the incision will be.

4. The most common problems after surgery are pneumonia, bleeding, infection, clotted blood (hematoma) at the surgery site, or a reaction to the anesthesia. In the first 48 hours after surgery, the most likely risks are bleeding or problems with heart or lungs.

Unit Nine

A. Translate the following sentences into Chinese.

1. 出血是可预防性损伤后死亡的主要原因，低血容量性休克是因为大量失血造成的。

2. 正常心音的存在可通过听诊确认。如果出现外出血，应该通过按压或手术来止血。

3. 指南将会从以往五年进行一次修改和更新调整为基于网络平台的持续更新。

4. 建议成人胸外按压幅度是至少 2 英寸（5 厘米），但不超过 2.4 英寸（6 厘米）。

B. Translate the following sentences into English.

1. The goal of the primary assessment is to rapidly identify potentially life-threatening conditions requiring immediate interventions.

2. The goal of most emergency medical services is to either provide treatment to those in need of urgent medical care, or arranging for timely removal of the patient to the next point of definitive care.

3. The recommended chest compression rate is 100 to 120/min (updated from at least 100/min).

4. The AHA adult Chain of Survival includes 2 chains: one for in-hospital and the other for out-of-hospital systems of care.

Unit Ten

A. Translate the following sentences into Chinese.

1. 你可能会发现，做出一些小的改变就能确保饮食的健康和平衡。

2. 为了避免疾病，《2005 年美国饮食指南》建议饮食中富含水果、蔬菜、全谷类和脱脂奶制品。

3. 因为免疫球蛋白 A 能够阻止吸收那些促成过敏发生的外来分子，所以母乳不会引起过敏。

4. 虽然母乳中的铁含量低于配方奶粉，但是母乳中大约 50% 铁可以被吸收，相比之下，高铁配方奶粉中仅有 7% 被吸收。

B. Translate the following sentences into English.

1. A client who cannot maintain proper nutrition because of poor teeth will have inadequate nutrition as a health care need.

2. Vitamin D plays an important role in preventing and curing cancer and heart disease.

3. Sometimes, people are not clear about what kinds of food are healthy, and what kinds of food may do harm to their health.

4. Part of the postpartum nurse's daily responsibility is to provide individual instruction and support to mothers who are under her care.

Unit Eleven

A. Translate the following sentences into Chinese.

1. 痴呆是一种慢性或进展性的综合征，患者会出现与正常衰老并不相同的认知功能退化（例如思维能力）。

2. 对家庭和照料者而言，身体、情感和经济等方面的压力非常巨大，因此需要来自健康、社会、财政和法律等体系的支持。

3. 社区健康护理是护理实践和公共健康实践的综合应用，可以促进和保持民众的健康。

4. 痴呆患者的家庭面临的问题非常复杂，因此压力巨大。除了健康问题，他们还面临着经济困难。

B. Translate the following sentences into English.

1. Worldwide, 47.5 million people have dementia, with just over half (58%) living in low- and middle-income countries.

2. The community health nurse's perspective on dementia will influence the nursing role and the level of care he or she provides to patient with dementia and their families.

3. Alzheimer's disease (AD) was named after Alois Alzheimer, a German doctor who found it in 1907. It accurately described the typical brain alterations related to morphological, neurochemical, and physiological dysfunction.

4. The symptoms include a decline in mental status involving changes in memory, language, praxis, mood, concentration, cooperation, thought process, and perception with progressive deterioration.

Unit Twelve

A. Translate the following sentences into Chinese.

1. 临终关怀是一种关于照护临终患者及其家属的理念和模式。

2. 通过治疗疼痛、其他症状以及心理和精神困扰，采用高超的沟通技巧确立护理目标，制订个性化治疗方案，并通过协调性照护，使安宁疗护（姑息护理）及其他与疾病相关的治疗在确诊之时即可一并提供。

3. 只要患者的医生和临终关怀团队确认生命有限，而且患者自愿放弃根治性治疗，就适于临终关怀干预项目。

4. 疼痛、易怒、呼吸困难、呼吸道分泌物、恶心和呕吐是患者临终前几天或数小时可能出现的最常见问题。其他一些症状也会出现，但某种程度上可能较轻，包括咳嗽、疲乏、发热，时有出血。

B. Translate the following sentences into English.

1. The complexity and severity of patients' condition lead to a hospital stay despite the willingness of family and friends to provide care at home.

2. Oral care is given by diluting the saline water or using 0.9% sodium chloride solution, three or four times a day.

3. During the dying process, patients' renal and liver function decline, decreasing metabolism and rate of drug clearance and leading to accumulation of dosages and drug toxicities.

4. Medications used for palliative patients include the use of non-opioid and opioid analgesics to relieve pain, anti-emetics for nausea, laxative to treat constipation, and sedative for delirium and restlessness.

Unit Thirteen

A. Translate the following sentences into Chinese.

1. 康复是一个动态的、以健康为导向的过程。它帮助患者或残障人员尽可能地恢复在生理、心理、精神、社会以及经济等方面的功能。

2. 康复的目的是让中风患者最大程度地恢复自理能力和工作能力。

3. 护理中风患者的护士有两个主要任务：尽可能控制中风导致的损伤，并确保康复计划的制订和实施。

4. 中风患者往往有复杂的康复需求，因此患者的进步和恢复各不相同。

B. Translate the following sentences into English.

1. Therapies and services used in rehabilitation depend on the individual needs.

2. The responsibility of nurses is to be closely involved in planning and implementing a program of rehabilitation in accordance with the patient's goals.

3. The need for rehabilitation runs through all age groups, though the types, levels, and goals of rehabilitation often differ.

4. Rehabilitation services are needed by more people than ever before because of advances in technology that save the lives of critically ill, injured, and disabled patients.

Unit Fourteen

A. Translate the following sentences into Chinese.

1. 因此，中医不仅可以辨病、治病、防病，而且同样重要的是，中医能够使健康、幸福和我们的生活和世界中的可持续性得到优化。

2. 中药在很多方面与西药相似，尽管中药强调的重点是促进阴阳的平衡。

3. 在治疗之前，医师应该向患者进行充分解释，以便消除对针灸的恐惧和焦虑。

4. 它们被直接运用在身体表面，通过施加外力来刺激身体，从而预防和治疗疾病。

B. Translate the following sentences into English.

1. The waxing and waning of *yin* and *yang* means that *yin* and *yang* oppose each other and yet depend on each other for existence, and they are not stagnant but in a dynamic state.

2. Preponderance of *yang* leads to hyper-function of the organism and heat manifestations, while preponderance of *yin* leads to hypo-function of the organism or endogenous cold. Deficiency of *yang* brings on symptoms of external cold, while deficiency of *yin* leads to endogenous heat.

3. Inquiry plays a very important role in TCM diagnosis, providing an important basis for defining *yin* or *yang*, interior or exterior, cold or heat, deficiency or excess of diseases.

4. Cupping is widely used to treat colds, respiratory tract infections, asthma, diarrhea, and other problems in the internal organs, and it has the function of relieving muscle spasms, stimulating blood circulation and enhancing human body immunity.

Unit Fifteen

NCLEX-RN® Practice Questions Set 1

1. Answer: C

The priority nursing action for a patient arriving at the ED in distress is always assessment of vital signs. This indicates the extent of physical compromise and provides a baseline by which to plan further assessment and treatment. A thorough medical history, including onset of symptoms, will be necessary and it is likely that an electrocardiogram will be performed as well, but these are not the first priority. Similarly, chest exam with auscultation may offer useful information after vital signs are assessed.

2. Answer: C

It is always critical that patients being discharged from the hospital take prescribed medications as instructed. In the case of antibiotics, a full course must be completed even after symptoms have resolved to prevent incomplete eradication of the organism and recurrence of infection. The patient should resume normal activities as tolerated, as well as a nutritious diet. Continued use of the incentive spirometer after discharge will speed recovery and improve lung function.

3. Answer: C

When a family member is dying, it is most helpful for nursing staff to provide a culturally sensitive environment to the degree possible within the hospital routine. In the Vietnamese culture, it is important that the dying be surrounded by loved ones and not left alone. Traditional rituals and foods are thought to ease the transition to the next life. When possible, allowing the family privacy for this traditional behavior is best for them and the patient. Answers A, B, and D are incorrect because they create unnecessary conflict with the patient and family.

4. Answer: A

The charge nurse planning assignments must consider the skills of the staff and the needs of the patients. The labor and delivery nurse who is not experienced with the needs of cardiac patients should be assigned to those with the least acute needs. The patient who is one-week post-operative and nearing discharge is likely to require routine care. A new patient admitted with suspected MI and scheduled for angiography would require continuous assessment as well as coordination of care that is best carried out by experienced staff. The unstable patient requires staff that can immediately identify symptoms and respond appropriately. A post-operative patient also requires close monitoring and cardiac experience.

5. Answer: B

Glucagon is given to treat insulin overdose in an unresponsive patient. Following Glucagon administration, the patient should respond within 15-20 minutes at which time oral carbohydrates should be given. Glucagon reverses rather than enhances or prolongs the effects of insulin. Lipoatrophy refers to the effect of repeated insulin injections on subcutaneous fat.

6. Answer: D

One gel pad should be placed to the right of the sternum, just below the clavicle and the other just left of the precordium, as indicated by the anatomic location of the heart. To defibrillate, the paddles are placed over the pads. Options A, B, and C are not consistent with the position of the heart and are therefore incorrect responses.

7. Answer: D

All of the statements are true. The gurgles and clicks described in the question represent normal bowel sounds, which vary with the phase of digestion. Intestinal obstruction causes the sounds to intensify as the normal flow is blocked by the obstruction. The swishing and buzzing sound of turbulent blood flow may be heard in the abdomen in the presence of abdominal aortic aneurism, for example, and should always be considered abnormal.

8. Answer: A

Emergency treatment following a chemical splash to the eye includes immediate irrigation with normal saline. The irrigation should be continued for at least 10 minutes. Fluorescein drops are used to check for scratches on the cornea due to their fluorescent properties and are not part of the initial care of a chemical splash, nor is patching the eye. Following irrigation, visual acuity will be assessed.

9. Answer: D

Post-surgical nursing assessment after hip replacement should be principally concerned with the risk of neurovascular complications and the development of infection. A temperature of 101.8 °F (38.7℃) postoperatively is higher than the low grade that is to be expected and should raise concern. Some pain during repositioning and following physical therapy is to be expected and can be managed with analgesics. A small amount of bloody drainage on the surgical dressing is a result of normal healing.

10. Answer: B

During a witnessed seizure, nursing actions should focus on securing the patient's safely and curtailing the seizure. Restraining the limbs is not indicated because strong muscle contractions could cause injury. A side-lying position with head flexed forward allows for drainage of secretions and prevents the tongue from falling back, blocking the airway. Rectal diazepam may be a treatment ordered by the physician, who should be notified of the seizure.

11. Answer: C

Emergency triage involves quick patient assessment to prioritize the need for further evaluation and care. Patients with trauma, chest pain, respiratory distress, or acute neurological changes are always classified number one priority. Though the patient with chest pain presented in the question recently ate a spicy meal and may be suffering from heartburn, he also may be having an acute myocardial infarction and require urgent attention. The patient with fever, headache and muscle aches (classic flu symptoms) should be classified as non-urgent. The patient with the foot injury may have sustained a sprain or fracture, and the limb should be x-rayed as soon as is practical, but the damage is unlikely to worsen if there is a delay. The child's chin laceration may need to be sutured but is also non-urgent.

12. Answer: C

Normal serum calcium is 8.5-10 mg/dL. The patient is hypocalcemic. Increased gastric motility, resulting in hyperactive (not hypoactive) bowel sounds, abdominal cramping and diarrhea is an indication of hypocalcemia. Numbness in hands and feet and muscle cramps are also signs of hypocalcemia. Positive Chvostek's sign refers to the sustained twitching of facial muscles following tapping in the area of the cheekbone and is a hallmark of hypocalcemia.

13. Answer: A

A patient on nasogastric suction is at risk of metabolic alkalosis as a result of loss of hydrochloric acid in gastric fluid. Of the answers given, only answer A (pH 7.52, PCO_2 54 mm Hg) represents alkalosis. Answer B is a normal blood gas. Answer C represents respiratory acidosis. Answer D is borderline normal with slightly low PCO_2.

14. Answer: A

The effect of Coumadin is to inhibit clotting. The next step is to check the PT and INR to determine the patient's anticoagulation status and risk of bleeding. Vitamin K is an antidote to Coumadin and may be used in a patient who is at imminent risk of dangerous bleeding. Preparation for transfusion, as described in option C, is only indicated in the case of significant blood loss. If lab results indicate an anticoagulation level that would place the patient at risk of excessive bleeding, the surgeon may choose to delay surgery and discontinue the medication.

15. Answer: A and B

Normal hemoglobin in adults is 12 - 16 g/dL. Total cholesterol levels of 200 mg/dL or below are considered normal. Total serum protein of 7g/dL and glycosylated hemoglobin A1c of 5.4% are both normal levels.

16. Answer: B

An IV site that is red, warm, painful and swollen indicates that phlebitis has developed and the line should be discontinued and restarted at another site. Pain on movement should be managed by maneuvers such as splinting the limb with an IV board or gently shifting the position of the catheter before making a decision to remove the line. An IV line that is running slowly may simply need flushing or repositioning. A hematoma at the site is likely a result of minor bleeding at the time of insertion and does not require discontinuation of the line.

17. Answer: D

Fluid overload occurs when the fluid volume infused over a short period is too great for the vascular system, causing fluid leak into the lungs. Symptoms include dyspnea, rapid respirations, and discomfort as in the patient described. Febrile non-hemolytic reaction results in fever. Symptoms of allergic transfusion reaction would include flushing, itching, and a generalized rash. Acute hemolytic reaction may occur when a patient receives blood that is incompatible with his blood type. It is the most serious adverse transfusion reaction and can cause shock and death.

18. Answer: B, C, and D

Uterine contractions typically become stronger and occur more closely together following amniotomy. The FHR is assessed immediately after the procedure and followed closely to detect changes that may indicate cord compression. The procedure itself is painless and results in the quick expulsion of amniotic fluid. Following amniotomy, cervical checks are minimized because of the risk of infection.

19. Answer: D

An infant discharged home with hyperbilirubinemia (newborn jaundice) should be placed in a sunny rather than dimLy lit area with skin exposed to help process the bilirubin. Frequent feedings will help to metabolize the bilirubin. A recheck of the serum bilirubin and a physical exam within 72 hours will confirm that the level is falling and the infant is thriving and is well hydrated. Signs of dehydration, including decreased urine output and skin changes, indicate inadequate fluid intake and will worsen the hyperbilirubinemia.

20. Answer: A

All infants under 1 year of age weighing less than 20 lbs. should be placed in a rear-facing infant car seat secured properly in the back seat. Infant car seats should never be placed in the front passenger seat. Infants should always be placed in an approved car seat during travel, even on that first ride home from the hospital.

NCLEX-RN® Practice Questions Set 2

1. Answer: C

Toddlers typically learn bowel control before bladder control, with boys often taking longer to complete toilet training than girls. Many children are not trained until 36 months and this should not cause concern. Later training is rarely caused by psychological factors and is much more commonly related to individual developmental maturity. Reprimanding the child will not speed the process and may be confusing.

2. Answer: C

Babies and toddlers should not fall asleep with bottles containing liquid other than plain water due to the risk of dental decay. Sugars in milk or juice remain in the mouth during sleep and cause caries, even in teeth that have not yet erupted. When water is substituted for milk or juice, babies will often lose interest in the bottle at night.

3. Answer: B

Infants under 6 months may not be able to sleep for long periods because their stomachs are too small to hold adequate nourishment to take them through the night. After 6 months, it may be helpful to let babies put themselves back to sleep after waking during the night, but not prior to 6 months. Infants should always be placed on their backs to sleep. Research has shown a dramatic decrease in sudden infant death syndrome (SIDS) with back sleeping. Eye contact and verbal engagement with infants are important to language development. The best diet for infants under 4 months of age is breast milk or infant formula.

4. Answer: A, B, and C

A daily bowel movement is not necessary if the patient is comfortable and the bowels move regularly. Moderate exercise, such as walking, encourages bowel health, as does generous water intake. A diet high in fiber is also helpful. Laxatives should be used as a last resort and should not be taken regularly. Over time, laxatives can desensitize the bowel and worsen constipation.

5. Answer: C

Rheumatic fever is caused by an untreated group A B hemolytic Streptococcus infection in the previous 2-6 weeks, confirmed by a positive antistreptolysin O titer. Rheumatic fever is characterized by a red rash over the trunk and extremities as well as fever and other symptoms.

6. Answer: A

Weight gain is an early symptom of congestive heart failure due to accumulation of fluid. When diuretic therapy is inadequate, one would expect an increase in blood pressure, tachypnea, and tachycardia to result.

7. Answer: B

The therapeutic serum level for Dilantin is 10-20 mcg/mL. A level of 4 mcg/mL is sub-therapeutic and may be caused by patient non-compliance or increased metabolism of the drug. A level of 15 mcg/mL is therapeutic. Choices C and D are expressed in mcg/dL, which is the incorrect unit of measurement.

8. Answer: D

Acetaminophen in even modestly large doses can cause serious liver damage that may result in death. Immediate evaluation of liver function is indicated with consideration of N-acetylcysteine administration as an antidote. Tinnitus is associated with aspirin overdose, not acetaminophen. Diarrhea and hypertension are not associated with acetaminophen.

9. Answer: B

Morphine sulfate can suppress respiration and respiratory reflexes, such as cough. Patients should be monitored regularly for these effects to avoid respiratory compromise. Morphine sulfate does not significantly affect urine output, heart rate, or body temperature.

10. Answer: C

Following triage, an x-ray should be performed to rule out fracture. Ice, not heat, should be applied to a recent sports injury. An elastic bandage may be applied and pain medication given once fracture has been excluded.

11. Answer: D

A moderate amount of serous drainage from a recent surgical site is a sign of normal healing. Purulent drainage would indicate the presence of infection. A soiled dressing should be changed to avoid bacterial growth and to examine the appearance of the wound. The surgical site is typically covered by gauze dressings for a minimum of 48-72 hours to ensure that initial healing has begun.

12. Answer: C

Impaired perfusion to the right lower arm as a result of a closed cast may cause neurovascular compromise and severe pain, requiring immediate cast removal. Itching under the cast is common and fairly benign. Neurovascular compromise in the arm would not cause pain in the shoulder, as perfusion there would not be affected. Impaired perfusion would cause the fingers to be cool and pale. Increased warmth would indicate increased blood flow or infection.

13. Answer: A

Physical activity and daily exercise can help to improve movement and decrease pain in osteoarthritis. Joint pain and stiffness are often at their worst during the early morning after several hours of decreased movement. Acetaminophen is a pain reliever, but does not have anti-inflammatory activity. Ibuprofen is a strong anti-inflammatory, but should always be taken with food to avoid GI distress.

14. Answer: D

Alendronate can cause significant gastrointestinal side effects, such as esophageal irritation, so it should not be taken if a patient must stay in supine position. It should be taken upon rising in the morning with 8 ounces of water on an empty stomach to increase absorption. The patient should not eat or drink for 30 minutes after administration and should not lie down. ACE inhibitors are not contraindicated with alendronate and there is no iodine allergy relationship.

15. Answer: C

Prophylactic use of antibiotics is not indicated to prevent Lyme disease. Antibiotics are used only when symptoms develop following a tick bite. Insect repellant should be used on skin and clothing when exposure is anticipated. Clothing should be designed to cover as much exposed area as possible to provide an effective barrier. Close examination of skin and hair can reveal the presence of a tick before a bite occurs.

16. Answer: D

Immunization is available for the prevention of some, but not all, specific diseases. This type of immunity is "acquired" by causing antibodies to form in response to a specific pathogen. Natural immunity is present at birth because the infant acquires maternal antibodies. Immunization, like all medication, cannot be risk-free and should be considered based on the risk of the disease in question.

17. Answer: B

The patient may be experiencing an anaphylactic reaction. The most urgent action is to maintain an airway, particularly with visible oral swelling, followed by the administration of epinephrine by subcutaneous injection. The physician will see the patient as soon as possible with the above actions underway. Oral diphenhydramine is indicated for mild allergic reactions and is not appropriate for anaphylaxis.

18. Answer: A, B, and D

ADHD in children is frequently treated with CNS stimulant medications, which increase focus and improve concentration. Children often experience insomnia, agitation, and decreased appetite. Sleepiness is not a side effect of stimulants.

19. Answer: D

Abnormal facial movements and tongue protrusion in a patient taking haloperidol is most likely due to tardive dyskinesia, an adverse reaction to the antipsychotic. Depression may occur along with schizophrenia and would be characterized by such symptoms as loss of affect, appetite and/or sleep changes, and anhedonia. These depressive changes and lack of volition are part of the negative symptoms of schizophrenia. Psychotic hallucinations may be visual or auditory but do not include abnormal movements.

20. Answer: B

Hypoglycemia in diabetes mellitus causes confusion, indicating the need for carbohydrates. Polydipsia, blurred vision, and polyphagia are symptoms of hyperglycemia.

A

accessibility [əkˌsesəˈbɪləti] *n.*	可及性；易接近；可以得到	Unit 12
accountability [əˌkaʊntəˈbɪləti] *n.*	有义务；有责任	Unit 1
acoustic [əˈkuːstɪk] *adj.*	听觉的	Unit 3
acupoint [ˈækjʊpɒɪnt] *n.*	穴位	Unit 14
acupuncture [ˈækjupʌŋktʃə(r)] *n.*	针刺疗法	Unit 5
acute [əˈkjuːt] *adj.*	急性的；敏锐的；激烈的	Unit 5
addiction [əˈdɪkʃən] *n.*	上瘾，沉溺；癖嗜	Unit 12
adversity [ədˈvɜːsəti] *n.*	逆境	Unit 13
advocacy [ˈædvəkəsɪ] *n.*	主张；拥护；辩护	Unit 1
aeration [ˌeəˈreɪʃn] *n.*	通气，充气	Unit 8
aesthetically [iːsˈθetɪkli; esˈθetɪkli] *adv.*	审美地；美学观点上地	Unit 1
afflicted [əˈflɪktɪd] *vt.*	折磨；使受痛苦；使苦恼	Unit 11
aggravate [ˈægrəveɪt] *vt.*	加重；使恶化；激怒	Unit 5
agitation [ˌædʒɪˈteɪʃn] *n.*	激动；易怒；烦乱	Unit 12
alleviation [əˌliːviˈeɪʃn] *n.*	减轻，缓解；镇痛剂	Unit 1
alveoli [ælˈviəlai] *n.*	肺泡，泡，腺泡	Unit 8
ambiguity [ˌæmbɪˈgjuːəti] *n.*	含糊；不明确；模棱两可的话	Unit 1
ambulatory [ˈæmbjələtəri] *adj.*	移动的，走动的	Unit 2
amiloride [əˈmɪlɑːraɪd] *n.*	［医］盐酸阿米洛利；氨氯吡脒	Unit 6
amiodarone [ˌæmɪoʊˈdæroʊn] *adj.*	胺碘酮的	Unit 6
analgesia [ˈænəlˈdʒiziə] *n.*	镇痛	Unit 8
analgesic [ˌænəlˈdʒiːzɪk] *adj. n.*	止痛的；止痛剂；［药］镇痛剂	Unit 2
anaphylactic [ˌænəfiˈlæktik] *adj.*	过敏性的；导致过敏的	Unit 8
anesthesia [ˌænɪsˈθiziə] *n.*	麻醉，麻木	Unit 8
anesthetic [ˌænɪsˈθetɪk] *n.*	麻醉剂；麻药	Unit 5
angina [ænˈdʒaɪnə] *n.*	心绞痛；咽峡炎；咽喉痛	Unit 4
anguish [ˈæŋgwɪʃ] *n.*	痛苦，苦恼；伤心，令人心酸	Unit 11
antiarrhythmic [ˌæntiəˈrɪðmɪk] *n.*	［医］抗心律失常的，抗心律不齐的；	

	抗心律失常药	Unit 6
antibiotic [ˌæntibaɪˈɒtɪk] n./adj.	抗生素；抗生的；抗菌的	Unit 6
around-the-clock	连续不断的，全天候的，日夜不停的	Unit 6
arrhythmia [eɪˈrɪðmɪə] n.	心律不齐	Unit 4
ascribe [əˈskraɪb] v.	归因于，归咎于	Unit 14
asthenia [əsˈθiːnɪə] n.	无力，衰弱	Unit 14
asthma [ˈæsmə] n.	气喘，支气管哮喘	Unit 8
atelectasis [ˌætɪˈlɛktəsɪs] n.	肺不张，肺膨胀不全	Unit 8
atheromatous [ˌæθəˈrɑmətəs] adj.	动脉粥样化的	Unit 4
audible [ˈɔːdəbl] adj.	听得见的	Unit 3
auscultation [ˌɔːskəlˈteɪʃn] n.	听诊	Unit 3
authority [ɔːˈθɒrəti] n.	权威；权力；当局	Unit 1
autonomy [ɔːˈtɒnəmi] n.	自治，自治权	Unit 1
auxiliary [ɔːgˈzɪliəri] adj.	辅助的；副的；附加的	Unit 1
axillary [ækˈsɪləri] adj.	腋窝的	Unit 4

B

ballottement [bæˈlɒtmənt] n.	冲击触诊法	Unit 3
bedridden [ˈbedrɪdn] adj.	卧床不起的	Unit 12
benzodiazepine [ˌbenzəʊdaɪˈeɪzɪpiːn] n.	苯二氮平类药物	Unit 12
bereavement [bɪˈriːvmənt] n.	丧友，丧亲；丧失	Unit 12
bicarbonate [ˌbaɪˈkɑːbənət] n.	碳酸氢盐；重碳酸盐	Unit 12
bile [baɪl] n.	胆汁	Unit 10
biopsy [ˈbaɪɒpsi] n.	活体组织检查	Unit 2
bisoprolol [baɪˈsɒprɒlɒl] n.	［医］比索洛尔〈β 受体阻滞药〉	Unit 6
bladder [ˈblædə(r)] n.	膀胱；囊；气泡；囊状物	Unit 7
boost [buːst] vt.	提高；促进；增加；改善	Unit 10
bowel [ˈbaʊəl] n.	肠；内部，最深处	Unit 7
bradycardia [ˌbrædɪˈkɑːdɪə] n.	心动过缓	Unit 4
bradypnea [bræˈdipniə] n.	呼吸过慢	Unit 4
breast [brest] n.	乳房；胸部	Unit 10
bronchitis [brɒŋˈkaɪtɪs] n.	支气管炎	Unit 14
bumetanide [bʌmetəˈnɪd] n.	［医］丁脲胺；布美他尼	Unit 6
butt [bʌt] v.	以头抵撞	Unit 14
bystander [ˈbaɪstændə(r)] n.	旁观者，看热闹的人	Unit 9

C

calcium [ˈkælsɪəm] n.	［化学］钙	Unit 2

cardiopulmonary [ˌkɑːdiəʊˈpʌlmənəri] *adj.*	心肺的	Unit 3
cardiovascular [ˌkɑːdiəʊˈvæskjələ(r)] *adj.*	心血管的	Unit 4
carvedilol [kɑːviːdɪˈlɒl] *n.*	［医］卡维地洛第三代 β 受体阻滞剂	Unit 6
casein [ˈkeɪsɪɪn] *n.*	［生化］酪蛋白；干酪素	Unit 10
catheterization [ˌkæθɪtəraɪˈzeɪʃən] *n.*	导管插入	Unit 7
cervical [ˈsəːvɪkl] *adj.*	颈的；子宫颈的	Unit 9
chaotic [keɪˈɒtɪk] *adj.*	混沌的；混乱的，无秩序的	Unit 13
chaplain [ˈtʃæplɪn] *n.*	牧师；专职教士	Unit 12
chemotherapy [kiːməʊˈθerəpi] *n.*	化学疗法；化学药物治疗	Unit 5
chlorothiazide [ˌklɔːrə(ʊ)ˈθaɪəzaɪd; ˈklɒ-] *n.*	［医］氯噻嗪；氯噻（一种利尿降压剂）	Unit 6
cholesterol [kəˈlestərɒl] *n.*	［生化］胆固醇	Unit 10
choreograph [ˈkɔriəgrɑːf] *vt.*	设计舞蹈动作；为……编舞	Unit 9
chronic [ˈkrɒnɪk] *adj.*	慢性的；长期的；习惯性的	Unit 5
clopidogrel [kˈləʊpɪdəgrəl] *n.*	［医］氯吡格雷（抑制血小板药物）； 克拉匹多	Unit 6
clot [klɒt] *n.*	凝块	Unit 13
cognitive [ˈkɒgnətɪv] *adj.*	认知的；认识的	Unit 11
collaborative [kəˈlæbəretɪv] *adj.*	合作的，协作的	Unit 1
collapse [kəˈlæps] *v.*	使倒塌，使崩溃	Unit 14
collateral [kəˈlætərəl] *n.*	络脉	Unit 14
commode [kəˈməʊd] *n.*	便桶	Unit 13
complication [ˌkɒmplɪˈkeɪʃn] *n.*	并发症	Unit 2
component [kəmˈpəʊnənt] *n.*	成分；组件	Unit 1
concentration [ˌkɒnsnˈtreɪʃn] *n.*	浓度，含量，专心，专注，集中，集结	Unit 6
confusion [kənˈfjuːʒn] *n.*	混淆；混乱；困惑	Unit 3
consciousness [ˈkɒnʃəsnəs] *n.*	知觉；觉悟；意识，观念；感觉	Unit 11
constipation [ˌkɒnstɪˈpeɪʃn] *n.*	便秘	Unit 5
constitution [ˌkɒnstɪˈtjuːʃn] *n.*	体格	Unit 14
contraindicate [ˌkɒntrəˈɪndɪkeɪt] *v.*	禁忌，显示不当	Unit 8
controversy [ˈkɒntrəvəːsi] *n.*	争论；论战；辩论	Unit 9
conversational [ˌkɒnvəˈseɪʃənl] *adj.*	会话的，谈话的；健谈的，善应酬的	Unit 11
convert [kənˈvɜːt] *vt.*	（使）转变；使皈依；兑换，换算	Unit 6
coordinate [kəʊˈɔːdɪneɪt] *v.*	协调，调整	Unit 14
coronary [ˈkɒrənri] *adj.*	冠状的，（心脏的）冠状动脉的	Unit 4
coumadin [kəˈmædɪn] *n.*	［医］香豆素；香豆定：苄丙酮香豆素钠 （sodium warfarin）制剂的商品名	Unit 6
creatinine [krɪˈætɪniːn] *n.*	［生化］肌酸酐	Unit 2
cuisine [kwɪˈziːn] *n.*	烹饪，烹调法	Unit 14
culprit [ˈkʌlprɪt] *n.*	问题的起因；罪犯；元凶	Unit 13
cultivation [ˌkʌltɪˈveɪʃn] *n.*	培养	Unit 14

D

debris ['debri:] *n.*	碎片，残骸	Unit 9
definitive [dɪ'fɪnətɪv] *adj.*	确定性的	Unit 9
delirium [dɪ'lɪrɪəm] *n.*	谵妄；精神错乱；发狂	Unit 12
delusion [dɪ'luːʒn] *n.*	妄想；错觉；欺骗；谬见	Unit 11
dementia [dɪ'menʃə] *n.*	［医］痴呆	Unit 11
dentist ['dentɪst] *n.*	牙科医生	Unit 2
descendent [dɪ'sendənt] *n.*	派生物	Unit 14
deterioration [dɪˌtɪərɪə'reɪʃn] *n.*	恶化；退化；变坏，堕落	Unit 11
diabetes [ˌdaɪə'biːtiːz] *n.*	糖尿病；多尿症	Unit 6
dialysis [ˌdaɪ'æləsɪs] *n.*	透析	Unit 2
diaphragm ['daɪəfræm] *n.*	横膈膜	Unit 3
diarrhea [ˌdaɪə'riə] *n.*	腹泻；痢疾	Unit 6
diastolic [ˌdaɪə'stɒlɪk] *adj.*	心脏舒张（期）的	Unit 4
dietitian [ˌdaɪə'tɪʃn] *n.*	营养师	Unit 2
differentiate [ˌdɪfə'renʃieɪt] *v.*	区分，区别	Unit 14
dilute [daɪ'l(j)uːt] *adj.& v.*	稀释的，淡的；稀释，冲淡	Unit 12
dimension [daɪ'menʃn; dɪ'menʃn] *n.*	方面；［数］维；尺寸	Unit 1
disharmony [dɪs'hɑːməni] *n.*	不调和，不融洽	Unit 14
disorder [dɪs'ɔːdə(r)] *n.*	（身体、精神的）失调；不适	Unit 2
disorientation [dɪsˌɔːriən'teɪʃn] *n.*	方向障碍；迷惑	Unit 11
dispensary [dɪ'spensəri] *n.*	药房，诊疗所	Unit 2
diuretic [ˌdaɪju'retɪk] *n.*	［医］利尿剂	Unit 6
drainage ['dreɪnɪdʒ] *n.*	排水，引流，排水道	Unit 8
Dullness ['dʌlnəs] *n.*	浊音	Unit 3
dynamic [daɪ'næmɪk] *adj.*	动态的；有活力的	Unit 13
dysfunction [dɪs'fʌŋkʃn] *n.*	机能障碍，机能失调	Unit 11
dyspnea [dɪsp'niːə] *n.*	呼吸困难	Unit 3
dyspnoea [dɪsp'niː ə] *n.*	呼吸困难	Unit 4

E

elasticity [ˌiːlæ'stɪsəti] *n.*	弹性，弹力	Unit 14
electrolyte [ɪ'lektrəlaɪt] *n.*	电解液，电解质	Unit 8
elicit [ɪ'lɪsɪt] *v.*	抽出；引出	Unit 3
eligible ['elɪdʒəbl] *adj.*	合格的，合适的；符合条件的	Unit 12
emergency [ɪ'mɜːdʒənsi] *n.*	急诊，意外	Unit 2
emphysema [ˌemfɪ'siːmə] *n.*	肺气肿	Unit 3
empirical [ɪm'pɪrɪkl] *adj.*	经验主义的，完全根据经验的	Unit 1

empower [ɪmˈpaʊə(r)] *vt.*　　　　　授权，允许；使能够　　　　　　　　　Unit 1

encapsulate [inˈkæpsjuleit] *vt.*　　封装　　　　　　　　　　　　　　　　Unit 9

encompass [ɪnˈkʌmpəs] *vt.*　　　　包含；包围，环绕　　　　　　　　　　Unit 1

endotracheal [ˌendəuˈtreikiəl] *adj.*　气管内的　　　　　　　　　　　　　Unit 9

enzyme [ˈenzaɪm] *n.*　　　　　　　［生化］酶　　　　　　　　　　　　Unit 6

epidemiological [ˌepɪˌdi:miəˈlɒdʒɪkl] *adj.*　流行病学的　　　　　　　　Unit 2

erythematosus [ˌɛriˌθi:məˈtəusəs] *n.& adj.*　全身性红斑狼疮；红斑的　　Unit 2

escalate [ˈeskəleɪt] *vt.*　　　　　使逐步升级，使逐步上升；乘自动梯上升　Unit 11

ethical [ˈeθɪkl] *adj.*　　　　　　伦理学的；道德的，伦理的；

　　　　　　　　　　　　　　　凭处方出售的　　　　　　　　　　　Unit 11

ethics [ˈeθɪks] *n.*　　　　　　　伦理学；伦理观；道德标准　　　　　Unit 1

exhaustion [ɪgˈzɔ:stʃən] *n.*　　　枯竭；耗尽；精疲力竭　　　　　　　Unit 5

exhaustive [ɪgˈzɔ:stɪv] *adj.*　　　详尽的，彻底的　　　　　　　　　　Unit 14

extraneous [ɪkˈstreɪnɪəs] *adj.*　　外部的　　　　　　　　　　　　　　Unit 3

extraordinarily [ɪkˈstrɔ:dnrəli] *adv.*　格外地，非凡地　　　　　　　　Unit 14

F

fatigue [fəˈtl:g] *n.*　　　　　　疲劳；疲乏　　　　　　　　　　　　Unit 3

feces [ˈfi:si:z] *n.*　　　　　　　粪；屎；渣滓　　　　　　　　　　　Unit 7

feeble [ˈfi:bl] *adj.*　　　　　　微弱的，虚弱的　　　　　　　　　　Unit 14

fiscal [ˈfɪskl] *adj.*　　　　　　　会计的，财政的　　　　　　　　　　Unit 1

forgo [fɔ:ˈgəu] *v.*　　　　　　　放弃；停止；对……断念　　　　　　Unit 12

furosemide [fjuˈrəusəmaɪd] *n.*　［医］呋喃苯胺酸；速尿灵（强效利尿剂）Unit 6

G

gastrointestinal [ˌgæstrəuɪnˈtestɪnl] *adj.*　胃肠的　　　　　　　　　　Unit 7

geriatric [ˌdʒerɪˈætrɪk] *adj.*　　老年医学的　　　　　　　　　　　　Unit 2

granulomatosis [ˈgrænjuˌləuməˈtəusis] *n.*　［医］肉芽肿病　　　　　　Unit 2

（复数 granulomatoses）

gym [dʒɪm] *n.*　　　　　　　　健身房　　　　　　　　　　　　　　Unit 13

gynecological [ˌgaɪnɪkəˈlɒdʒɪkəl] *adj.*　妇科（学）的　　　　　　　　Unit 2

H

hamper [ˈhæmpɚ] *vt.& n.*　　　妨碍；束缚；使困累；阻碍物　　　　Unit 12

hematuria [ˌhi:məˈtjuərɪə] *n.*　血尿；血尿症　　　　　　　　　　　Unit 7

hemodynamic [ˌhi:məudaiˈnæmik] *adj.*　血液动力学的　　　　　　　　Unit 9

hemoptysis [hɪˈmɒptɪsɪs] *n.*　　咳血，咯血　　　　　　　　　　　　Unit 4

hemorrhage ['hɛmərɪdʒ] n.	出血	Unit 9
hemothorax [ˌhi:mə'θɔ:ræks] n.	血胸	Unit 9
hernia ['hɜ·nɪə] n.	疝，疝气	Unit 8
holism ['həʊlɪzəm] n.	整体论	Unit 14
holistic [hə'lɪstɪk] adj.	整体的；全盘的	Unit 1
hospice [' hɒspɪs] n.	收容所；旅客招待所；救济院	Unit 12
hydralazine [haɪ'dræləzɪn] n.	［医］阿普利素灵，肼屈嗪	Unit 6
hydrochlorothiazide ['haɪdrəʊˌklɔ:rə'θaɪəzaɪd] n.		
	［医］氢氯噻嗪；二氢氯噻；双氢克尿噻	Unit 6
hyperpyrexia [ˌhaɪpəpaɪ'reksɪə] n.	高热，体温过高	Unit 4
hyperresonance [ˌhaɪpə'rezənəns] n.	过清音	Unit 3
hypertension [ˌhaɪpə'tenʃn] n.	高血压	Unit 4
hyperthermia [ˌhaɪpə'θɜ:mɪə] n.	过高热，极高热	Unit 4
hypoglycemia [ˌhaipəuglai'si:mɪə] n.	低血糖症；血糖过低	Unit 9
hypotension [haɪpə(ʊ)'tenʃ(ə)n] n.	低血压	Unit 4
hypothermia [ˌhaɪpə'θɜ:mɪə] n.	体温过低	Unit 4
hypoxia [haɪ'pɒksɪə] n.	低氧；组织缺氧；氧不足	Unit 3

I

ibuprofen [ˌaɪbju:'prəʊfen] n.	［医］布洛芬，异丁苯丙酸（抗炎镇痛药）	Unit 6
ignite [ɪg'naɪt] v.	点火；燃烧	Unit 14
illuminate [ɪ'lu:mɪneɪt] v.	阐明；照亮	Unit 3
immobilization [iˌməʊbəlai'zeiʃn] n.	固定	Unit 9
immunodeficiency [ɪˌmju:nəʊdɪ'fɪʃnsi] n.	免疫缺陷	Unit 7
immunoglobulin [ˌɪmjʊnəʊ'glɒbjʊlɪn] n.	免疫球蛋白；免疫血球素	Unit 10
implement ['ɪmplɪm(ə)nt] vt.	实施，执行；使生效	Unit 1
incapacitate [ˌɪnkə'pæsɪteɪt] vt.	使无能力；使不能	Unit 5
incentive [ɪn'sɛntɪv] adj.	激励的，刺激的	Unit 8
inception [ɪn'sepʃn] n.	开端，初期	Unit 14
incision [ɪn'sɪʒn] n.	切口，刀口	Unit 8
incubate ['ɪŋkjubeɪt] n.	（卵）被孵化；逐渐形成；潜伏（在体内）	Unit 7
indapamide [ɪndəpə'maɪd] n.	［医］吲达帕胺利尿降压药	Unit 6
infant ['ɪnfənt] n.	婴儿；幼儿	Unit 10
infarction [ɪn'fɑ:kʃn] n.	梗死；梗死形成	Unit 4
infection [ɪn'fekʃn] n.	感染；传染；影响；传染病	Unit 7
inheritance [ɪn'herɪtəns] n.	继承；遗传；遗产	Unit 11
inhibitor [ɪn'hɪbɪtə(r)] n.	抑制剂，抑制者；抗老化剂	Unit 6
insidious [ɪn'sɪdɪəs] adj.	阴险的；隐伏的，潜在的	Unit 11
insomnia [ɪn'sɒmnɪə] n.	失眠症，失眠	Unit 7

inspection [ɪn'spekʃn] n.	视诊	Unit 3
institution [ˌɪnstɪ'tuːʃən] n.	公共机构，协会，慈善机构	Unit 2
insulate ['ɪnsjuleɪt] v.	隔离，使孤立	Unit 14
integral ['ɪntɪɡrəl] adj.	完整的；不可或缺的	Unit 13
interact [ˌɪntər'ækt] v.	互相影响，互相作用	Unit 14
interference [ɪntə'fɪərəns] n.	干扰；干涉	Unit 5
intermittent [ˌɪntə'mɪtənt] adj.	间歇的；断断续续的；间歇性	Unit 5
intern ['ɪntɜːn] n.	实习医师	Unit 2
interstitial [ˌɪntə'stɪʃl] adj.	间质的；空隙的	Unit 2
intervention [ˌɪntə'venʃn] n.	干预，介入	Unit 5
intestine [ɪn'testɪn] n.	肠；肠管	Unit 10
intravenously [ɪntrə'viːnəsli] adv.	静脉注射地；通过静脉	Unit 5
intuition [ˌɪntjuː'ɪʃn] n.	直觉	Unit 1
irritability [ɪrɪtə'bɪləti] n.	过敏性；易怒；兴奋性	Unit 5
ischemic [ɪs'kimɪk] adj.	缺血性的	Unit 13

J

jaundice ['dʒɔːndɪs] n.	黄疸；偏见；乖僻；使患黄疸	Unit 7
judgement ['dʒʌdʒmənt] n.	评价，判断；判决；意见；见识	Unit 11

L

lactose ['læktəʊs] n.	［化］乳糖	Unit 10
larynx ['lærɪŋks] n.	胸膜；肋膜	Unit 3
legume ['leɡjuːm; lɪ'ɡjuːm] n.	豆类；豆科植物；豆荚	Unit 10
lettuce ['letɪs] n.	［园艺］生菜；莴苣	Unit 10
lymph [lɪmf] n.	淋巴；淋巴液	Unit 3

M

malignant [mə'lɪɡnənt] adj.	恶性的；有害的	Unit 8
maneuver [mə'nʊvə-] n.	操作	Unit 8
manikin ['mænɪkɪn] n.	人体模型；侏儒	Unit 9
massage ['mæsɑːʒ] n.	按摩	Unit 14
maternal [mə'tɜːnl] adj.	母亲的；母性的；母系的	Unit 10
medication administration	给药	Unit 6
medication errors	用药差错	Unit 6
meditation [ˌmedɪ'teɪʃn] n.	沉思，深思	Unit 14
meridian [mə'rɪdiən] n.	经脉	Unit 14

metabolic [ˌmɛtə'bɒlɪk] adj.	新陈代谢的，代谢作用的，代谢的	Unit 8
metastatic [ˌmetə'stætɪk] adj.	转移性的；转移的	Unit 5
metolazone ['miːtɔlæzəun] n.	［医］美托拉宗；甲苯喹唑磺胺	Unit 6
metoprolol [mɪ'tɑːprəlɒl] n.	［医］美托洛尔	Unit 6
microscopic [ˌmaɪkrə'skɒpɪk] adj.	显微镜的，用显微镜可见的；	
	微小的，细微的	Unit 7
midwife ['mɪdwaɪf] n.	助产士	Unit 2
milestone ['maɪlstəun] n.	里程碑；划时代的事件	Unit 13
mitigable ['mɪtɪɡəbl] adj.	可缓和的；可减轻的	Unit 12
mitral ['maɪtrəl] adj.	二尖瓣的	Unit 3
monkshood ['mʌŋkshʊd] n.	舟形乌头	Unit 14
morphological [ˌmɔːfə'lɒdʒɪkl] adj.	形态学的；形态的	Unit 11
mourning ['mɔːnɪŋ] n.	哀痛；服丧	Unit 12
moxibustion [ˌmɒksɪ'bʌstʃ(ə)n] n.	艾灸	Unit 14
mucous ['mjuːkəs] adj.	黏液的；分泌黏液的	Unit 7
murmur ['mɜˑrmər] n.	低语；杂音	Unit 3
myoclonus [ˌmaɪə(ʊ)'kləunəs] n.	肌阵挛	Unit 12

N

naproxen [nə'prɒksɛn] n.	萘普生；甲氧萘丙酸	Unit 6
nasal ['neɪzl] adj.	鼻的	Unit 3
nephritis [nɪ'fraɪtɪs] n.	肾炎	Unit 2
nephropathy [nə'frɒpəθi] n.	［泌尿］肾病	Unit 2
neurochemical [ˌnjʊərəʊ'kemɪkəl] n.	影响神经系统的化学物质	Unit 11
neuromuscular [ˌnjʊərəʊ'mʌskjʊlər] adj.	神经肌肉的	Unit 3
normalise ['nɔːməlaɪz] v.	（使）正常化；（使）恢复友好状态	Unit 12
numerical [njuː'merɪkl] adj.	数值的；数字的；用数字表示的	Unit 5

O

obstetric [əb'stetrɪk] adj.	产科（学）的	Unit 2
oncological [ɑnkə'lɒdʒikl] n.	肿瘤学	Unit 2
ongoing ['ɒngəʊɪŋ] adj.	不间断的；进行的	Unit 13
ophthalmoscope [ɒp'θælməskəup] n.	检眼镜	Unit 3
opioid ['əʊpɪɔɪd] n.	鸦片样物质；类鸦片	Unit 5
optimal ['ɒptɪməl] adj.	最佳的；最理想的	Unit 5
optimization [ˌɒptɪmaɪ'zeɪʃən] n.	最佳化，最优化	Unit 1
optimize ['ɒptɪmaɪz] v.	使最优化；使完善	Unit 14
organism ['ɔːɡənɪzəm] n.	有机物，有机体；生物	Unit 7

oriented ['ɔ:rɪentɪd] *adj.*	导向的；定向的；以……为方向的	Unit 13
originate [əˈrɪdʒɪneɪt] *v.*	发源，发生	Unit 14
orthopedic [ˌɔ:θəˈpi:dɪk] *adj.*	整形外科的	Unit 2
over-the-counter [əʊvəðə ˈkaʊntə(r)] *adj.*	［医］非处方药的	Unit 5
overwhelming [ˌoʊvərˈwelmɪŋ] *adj.*	势不可挡的，压倒一切的；巨大的	Unit 11

P

painkiller ['peɪnkɪlə(r)] *n.*	止痛药	Unit 5
palliative ['pælɪətɪv] *n.&adj.*	缓和剂；姑息的手段；缓和的	Unit 12
palpation [pælˈpeɪʃn] *n.*	触诊	Unit 3
pancreatic [ˌpæŋkrɪˈætɪk] *adj.*	胰的；胰腺的	Unit 12
paracetamol [pærəˈsi:təmɒl] *n.*	［药］扑热息痛	Unit 12
paralysis [pəˈræləsɪs] *n.*	麻痹；无力；停顿	Unit 12
paralyzed ['pærəˌlaɪzd] *adj.*	瘫痪的	Unit 13
parenteral [pəˈrent(ə)r(ə)l] *adj.*	肠胃外的，不经肠的，非肠道的；注射用药物的	Unit 6
pasta ['pæstə] *n.*	意大利面食；面团	Unit 10
pastoral ['pɒstərəl] *adj.*	牧人的；田园生活的；乡村的	Unit 8
patent ['pætnt] *adj.*	开放的；未闭的；不阻塞的	Unit 3
pathogen ['pæθədʒən] *n.*	病菌；病原体	Unit 7
pathology [pəˈθɒlədʒi] *n.*	病理（学）	Unit 12
pediatric [ˌpidɪˈætrɪk] *adj.*	儿科的	Unit 2
perception [pəˈsepʃn] *n.*	知觉；看法；洞察力	Unit 1
percussion [pəˈkʌʃn] *n.*	叩诊	Unit 3
pericardiocentesis ['periˌkɑ:dɪəʊsenti:sis] *n.*	心包穿刺术	Unit 9
peripheral [pəˈrɪfərəl] *adj.*	外围的；周边的	Unit 9
perspective [pəˈspektɪv] *n.*	观点，视角；远景	Unit 1
pharmacist ['fɑ:məsɪst] *n.*	药剂师	Unit 2
pharynx ['færɪŋks] *n.*	咽	Unit 3
physician [fɪˈzɪʃn] *n.*	医师，内科医师	Unit 2
pilgrim ['pɪlgrɪm] *n.*	朝圣者；漫游者	Unit 12
placenta [pləˈsentə] *n.*	胎盘	Unit 7
pleura ['plʊrə] *n.*	喉；喉头	Unit 3
pneumonia [njuˈməʊnɪə] *n.*	肺炎	Unit 8
pneumothorax [ˌnju:məʊˈθɔ:ræks] *n.*	气胸	Unit 9
potassium [pəˈtæsɪəm] *n.*	［化学］钾	Unit 2
poultry ['pəʊltri] *n.*	家禽；家禽肉	Unit 10
practitioner [prækˈtɪʃənə(r)] *n.*	开业医生，从业者	Unit 2
praxis ['præksɪs] *n.*	行为；实践；习题	Unit 11

precaution [prɪˈkɔːʃn] n.	预防措施，预防，防备，警惕	Unit 6
predispose [ˈpriːdɪˈspəʊz] vt.	预先处置；使……偏向于	Unit 3
pregnancy [ˈpregnənsi] n.	怀孕，妊娠	Unit 7
prescription [prɪˈskrɪpʃn] n.	处方	Unit 5
print out [ˈprɪntaʊt] n.	（电脑）打印件	Unit 6
prognosis [prɒgˈnəʊsɪs] n.	预后；预知	Unit 2
prominent [ˈprɒmɪnənt] adj.	著名的；突出的，杰出的；突起的	Unit 11
prompts [prɒmpts] n.	［计］提示	Unit 9
prophylaxis [ˌprɒfəˈlæksɪs] n.	预防；预防法	Unit 7
protein [ˈprəʊtiːn] n.	蛋白质	Unit 10
prothrombin [prəʊˈθrɒmbɪn] n.	凝血酶原	Unit 8
psychiatrist [saɪˈkaɪətrɪst] n.	精神病专家，精神病医师	Unit 2
psychologist [saɪˈkɒlədʒɪst] n.	心理学家	Unit 2
psychomotor [ˌsaɪkəʊˈməʊtə] adj.	精神运动的	Unit 11
purulent [ˈpjʊərələnt] adj.	脓的；含脓的	Unit 7

Q

quantify [ˈkwɒntɪfaɪ] vt.	量化；为……定量；确定数量	Unit 5

R

radiate [ˈreɪdieɪt] vi.	辐射；从中心向各方伸展	Unit 5
radiographer [ˌreɪdɪˈɒgrəfə] n.	放射科技师	Unit 2
radiographic [ˌreɪdɪəʊˈgræfɪk] adj.	射线照相术的	Unit 4
radiotherapy [reɪdɪəʊˈθerəpi] n.	放射治疗	Unit 5
recoil [riˈkɔil] n./vi.	畏缩；弹回；反作用	Unit 9
rectally [ˈrɛktli] adv.	直肠给药地	Unit 5
recumbent [rɪˈkʌmbənt] adj.	斜倚的；休息的	Unit 14
rehabilitation [ˌriːəˌbɪlɪˈteɪʃn] n.	康复（医学）	Unit 2
relinquish [rɪˈlɪŋkwɪʃ] vt.	放弃；放手	Unit 12
resonance [ˈrezənəns] n.	清音	Unit 3
respiratory [ˈrespərətri] adj.	呼吸的，呼吸用的	Unit 7
respite [ˈrespaɪt] n.	延期；（死刑）缓期执行；使休息	Unit 11
resuscitation [riˌsʌsiˈteiʃn] n.	复苏；复兴；复活	Unit 9
retinal [ˈretɪnl] adj.	视网膜的	Unit 13
retrieve [riˈtriːv] vt.	恢复；重新得到	Unit 9
rhythm [ˈrɪðəm] n.	［医］节律，规律；［乐］节拍；［艺］调和	Unit 6
rinse [rɪns] v. & n.	漱口；冲洗；漂净	Unit 12

S

saliva [sə'laɪvə] *n.*	唾液，口水	Unit 7
secretion [sɪ'kriːʃn] *n.*	分泌，分泌物；藏匿；隐藏	Unit 7
semen ['siːmən] *n.*	精液；精子	Unit 7
seven rights	七对	Unit 6
signify ['sɪgnɪfaɪ] *vt.*	表示；意味；预示	Unit 1
sophisticated [sə'fɪstɪkeɪtɪd] *adj.*	复杂的；精致的；富有经验的	Unit 12
specialize ['speʃəlaɪz] *v.*	专业化，专门化	Unit 2
specula ['spekjʊlə] *n.*	反射镜；诊视镜	Unit 3
spinal ['spaɪnl] *adj.*	脊髓的，脊柱的	Unit 8
spirometer [ˌspaɪ'rɒmɪtɚ] *n.*	呼吸量计，肺活量计	Unit 8
spirometry [spai'rɔmitri] *n.*	呼吸量测定法	Unit 8
spironolactone [ˌspaɪrənə(ʊ)'læktəʊn] *n.*	［医］安体舒通；螺内酯；螺旋内酯甾酮（一种利尿药）	Unit 6
splint [splɪnt] *n.*	夹板；薄木条	Unit 8
spondylosis [spɒndɪ'ləʊsɪs] *n.*	椎关节强硬	Unit 12
syringe [sɪ'rɪndʒ] *n.*	注射器	Unit 6
staff [staːf] *n.*	医务人员，工作人员	Unit 2
stakeholder ['steɪkhəʊldə(r)] *n.*	利益相关者；赌金保管者	Unit 9
statins [s'teɪtɪnz] *n.*	［医］他汀类药物	Unit 6
stenosis [stɪ'nəʊsɪs] *n.*	（器官）狭窄	Unit 4
sterile ['steraɪl] *adj.*	不生育的，不能生殖的；无菌的，消过毒的	Unit 7
steroid ['stɪɛrɔɪd] *n.*	类固醇	Unit 8
stethoscope ['steθəskəʊp] *n.*	听诊器	Unit 3
sthenia [sθɪ'naɪə] *n.*	强壮	Unit 14
stigmatization [ˌstɪgmətaɪ'zeɪʃn] *n.*	污名化；烙印化；描绘	Unit 11
stridor ['straɪdə] *n.*	喘鸣	Unit 4
stroke [strəʊk] *n.*	中风	Unit 13
subservient [səb'sɜːvɪənt] *adj.*	屈从的	Unit 1
substitute ['sʌbstɪtjuːt] *n.*	替代品；代用品；代替者	Unit 10
superintendent [ˌsupərɪn'tendənt] *n.*	院长，负责人	Unit 2
surgeon ['sɜːdʒən] *n.*	外科医生	Unit 2
sustainability [səˌsteɪnə'bɪləti] *n.*	持续性	Unit 14
swelling ['swelɪŋ] *n.*	肿胀；膨胀；增大	Unit 3
swollen ['swəʊlən] *adj.*	肿胀的；浮肿的	Unit 2
syndrome ['sɪndrəʊm] *n.*	综合征，综合症状，典型表现	Unit 11
systolic [ˌsɪ'stɒlɪk] *adj.*	心脏收缩（期）的	Unit 4

T

tachycardia [ˌtækɪˈkɑːdɪə] *n.*	心动过速	Unit 4
tachypnea [ˌtækɪpˈnɪə] *n.*	呼吸促迫，呼吸急促	Unit 4
tamponade [ˌtæmpəˈneid] *n.*	填塞	Unit 9
taurine [ˈtɔːriːn] *n.*	［化］牛磺酸，氨基乙磺酸	Unit 10
taxonomy [tækˈsɔnəmi] *n.*	分类学；分类法	Unit 9
testimony [ˈtestɪməni] *n.*	证词；证言	Unit 13
therapist [ˈθerəpɪst] *n.*	治疗师	Unit 2
thoracic [θoˈræsɪk] *adj.*	胸的，胸廓的	Unit 8
thoracostomy [ˌθorəˈkɑstəmi] *n.*	胸廓造口术	Unit 9
three checks	三查	Unit 6
thrill [θrɪl] *v.*	颤抖；震颤	Unit 3
thromboplastin [ˌθrombəˈplæstɪn] *n.*	促凝血酶原激酶	Unit 8
thyroid [ˈθaɪrɔɪd] *n.*	甲状腺	Unit 3
tomography [təˈmɔgrəfi] *n.*	X 线断层摄影术	Unit 9
tonsillar [ˈtaːnslə] *adj.*	扁桃体（腺）的	Unit 7
torasemide [tərəˈsemaɪd] *n.*	［医］胺吡磺异丙脲；间甲苯胺吡啶璜酰异丙脲；托拉塞米	Unit 6
tramp [træmp] *v.*	践踏，踩	Unit 14
treatise [ˈtriːtɪs] *n.*	专著；论述	Unit 14
triamterene [tˈrɪəmtəriːn] *n.*	［医］氨苯蝶啶；三氨蝶呤	Unit 6
triglyceride [traɪˈglɪsəraɪd] *n.*	［化］甘油三酯	Unit 10
tympanic [tɪmˈpænɪk] *adj.*	鼓膜的	Unit 4
tympany [ˈtɪmpəni] *n.*	鼓音	Unit 3

U

urinalysis [jʊərɪˈnælɪsɪs] *n.*	尿液分析	Unit 8
urinalysis [jʊrɪˈnælɪsɪs] *n.*	尿分析，验尿	Unit 7
utilize [ˈjuːtəlaɪz] *v.*	利用	Unit 14

V

vaginal [vəˈdʒaɪnl] *adj.*	阴道的	Unit 3
veterans [ˈvetərənz] *n.*	退伍军人；经验丰富的人；老兵	Unit 11
vibratory [ˈvaɪbrəˌtəri] *adj.*	振动的	Unit 3
vision [ˈvɪʒn] *n.*	视力	Unit 13

Y

yogurt ['jɒgət] *n.* 酸奶酪；[食品] 酸乳 Unit 10

Z

zidovudine [zɪ'dovjʊˌdin] *adj.* 齐多夫定；叠氮胸苷；叠氮胸腺 Unit 7

Appendix 3
Video and Audio Scripts

Unit One Nursing Today (Audio)

Part I Listening & Speaking
Task 1 Listening

A Nurse's Diary

Why choose geriatric nursing as a profession? This is a question which was asked of me many times during the course of my career as a nurse in long-term care. It isn't always an easy one to answer. Most people's concept of the "nursing home" nurse is that of a person who does not enjoy the respect given to other members of the healthcare profession, because many people do not see us as being "real" nurses. However, the reality of the situation is that some people discharged from hospitals are much sicker than they were before, and much more in need of assistance.

I began my first job in long-term care at the age of 17, as a nursing assistant. I have always enjoyed being around the elderly, and this is probably the primary reason I love being a "nursing home" nurse. The opportunity to really "connect" and build relationships with your patients is not something which is often found in the hospital setting, where patients stay only for a few days. There is a real challenge which comes along with taking care of someone for a few months or years as opposed to a few days. This challenge comes from trying to meet the patients' emotional needs as well as the physical needs, to provide a comfortable, "homelike" environment for the person, and to provide support, encouragement, and education for the patient's family members. The rewards received from meeting the challenge are significant, and are probably the major reason that those of us in long-term care stay in the profession. When I look back on my career, many years from now, the things which I remember will not be how hard I worked, or what technical skills I was able to perform successfully. The memories which stay with me will be those of someone's face lightening up when I entered the room, the time when I laughed and cried with my patients or their families; the batch of cookies made for me by a patient's daughter in gratitude for my care of her mother. These are the things which make my job worthwhile, and the reason I look forward to going to work each day.

Unit Two Admitting and Discharging a Patient (Video)

Part I Listening & Speaking
Task 1 Listening

(1)

Nurse: Mrs. Jones? Mrs. Tammy Jones?

Patient: Yes.

Nurse: Hi—my name is Linda, I'm one of the nurses from the Emergency Department, I'm going to bring you back to your room. Have a seat right here.

Patient: Okay.

Nurse: I'm really sorry you're not feeling well today. It says on your chart you're having a cough and shortness of breath?

Patient: Yes.

Nurse: Do you mind putting those foot rests in? Would you like to come with me ma'am? Okay, is that okay with you, Tammy?

Patient: Yes.

Nurse: Okay.

Patient: She's my sister, she can come with me.

Nurse: Perfect. We'll just bring you to your room right now.

Nurse: This is your room. This is room six Mrs. Jones, we're going to bring you in right here. And we'll get you undressed.

(2)

Nurse: Dawn, this is Mrs. Jones, and I'm bringing here from the ER.

Nurse 2: Mrs. Jones, you're now in room 375B.

Patient: Okay.

Nurse: Dawn is going to be your nurse. She's one of our most experienced nurses. I'm going to be going over your report on what we did in the emergency department, as far as your treatment plan and your diagnosis. And Dawn, she is here with a diagnosis of pneumonia, and Dr. Brown is her admission physician.

Nurse 2: Okay. Hi, Mrs. Jones.

Patient: Hi.

Nurse 2: Again, I am Dawn Sell and I'll be the one taking care of you today up here in room 375.Is it okay if I call you Tammy?

Patient: Yes, Tammy's fine.

Nurse 2: Okay, I'm Dawn.

Patient: Okay.

Nurse: So Dawn, Mrs. Jones, sorry Tammy, presented to the emergency department, with a cough of about 2 to 3 days (patient actually said 3 weeks) duration, nonproductive. She's a nonsmoker, low grade fever of 100.1. Her X-ray on exam in the ER shows a right lower lobe infiltrate. Our treatment plan had been to try and get her home, but her O_2 saturations on admission were 92%, she increased quite well with 4 liters of oxygen. But when we ambulated her in the emergency department on room air, her oxygen kept dropping to 92%. The ER physician contacted Dr. Brown, her doctor, and they felt her treatment plan would best benefit her with admission, with updraft Ventolin aerosol treatments every 4 to 6 hours, and some IV antibiotic therapy. Her white (blood) count was 10.7 in the emergency department. And her blood cultures currently are pending.

Nurse 2: What O_2 is she on now?

Nurse: Right now she is on 3 liters. She is doing quite well on 3 liters.

Nurse 2: Okay—all right.

Nurse: Okay. Her last dose of Levaquin, actually her initial dose of Levaquin was at noon, and it is prescribed daily.

Nurse 2: Okay. Looks like her saline lock is here in her left forearm. What size is it?

Nurse: That's a number 20 gauge in her arm.

Nurse 2: Okay. And it flushed fine?

Nurse: And it flushed fine.

Nurse 2: After Levaquin. Okay.

Nurse: Uh huh. Her vital signs, she's 98.7 currently. That's after a gram of Tylenol in the emergency department.

Nurse 2: Do you remember, or can you tell me when you last gave the Tylenol?

Nurse: Yes, at 11: 30.

Nurse 2: 11: 30. Okay.

Nurse: 11: 30 a.m. Her heart rate is 88, normal sinus rhythm, her EKG was within normal limits in the emergency department.

Nurse 2: Okay.

Nurse: Blood pressure is 120 over 70. As you can see she's doing well on the 3 liters of oxygen. She's 97% (O_2 saturation).

Nurse 2: Okay.

Nurse: Other than that, on the treatment plan we hope to get her home quite quickly, see if we can get her to discharge in the next 24 to 48 hours. That's our plan.

Nurse 2: Okay. When is she due for her respiratory treatment? Her Ventolin?

Nurse: Her last treatment was at noon.

Nurse 2: And it's every 4 to 6?

Nurse: It's every 4 to 6 hours so I believe that would be approximately 4 p.m.

Nurse 2: Okay.

Nurse: Okay. She complained of no pain while in the emergency department, but then after the aerosol therapy she had a headache. I did call Dr. Brown on the phone and asked him if she could have an order for something for her headache. He did order Norco, 5 milligrams that she can have every 4 to 6 hours. I did repeat that and verify that with Dr. Brown on the phone, and so there is a written

verbal order on the chart for that Norco. We did give that at 12: 30, just before we brought her up
　　to the floor.

Nurse 2: Okay. How's your headache? Did it help?

Patient: Yes, it did help. It's better.

Unit Three Health Assessment / Unit Four Clinical Observation (Video)

Part I　Listening & Speaking
Task 1　Listening

Narrator: In the following video clip please note that the nurse did the following:

■ Gave attention to patient comfort. Verified the patient identity by checking the name band and
asking the patient's name and birth date. Looked at the patient while asking health history questions.
Performed a Health Assessment.

■ Assessed the vital signs using the 2 step method which is recommended by the American Heart
Association

■ Checked the pulse oximeter reading

■ Warned the patient about possible discomfort

■ Thanked the patient

■ Give reasons for the cardiac monitor

■ Notice the nurse asked the patient, "May I examine your chest?"

The nurse also completed a medication reconciliation to verify home medications.

The nurse encouraged confidence in the physician, saying to the patient "Dr. Lynn has worked here
in the emergency room for 17 years."

Nurse 1: Heather is coming in to help me because we're going to work the two of us here. Thank you for
　　covering your mouth—thank you very much. And get you settled here and just find out what's
　　going on so that we can help you. Okay?

Nurse 2: Hi, I'm Heather, I'm another nurse. I'm going to go ahead and raise the head of your bed if that
　　will make you a little bit more comfortable.

Patient: Okay.

Nurse 2: All right. You want covered up?

Patient: Yes.

Nurse 2: All right. Would you like a Kleenex for your cough?

Patient: Thank you.

Nurse 2: You're very welcome.

Patient: Tammy Jones—10263.

Nurse 2: And are you allergic to anything?

Patient: Penicillin.

Nurse 2: Okay. I have a special red bracelet for you that will just notify all of us that you do have an
　　allergy.

Nurse 1: Mrs. Jones, I've introduced myself. It's Linda, I'm going to go through some of the questions about your complaints that you have today and your symptoms.

Patient: Okay.

Nurse 1: Okay. How long have you been sick, Mrs. Jones?

Patient: About 3 weeks.

Nurse 1: About 3 weeks—okay. You're having a cough, what your main complaint was when you came in?

Patient: Yes, cough and short of breath.

Nurse 1: Okay. With your cough, is it productive at all? Are you bringing up any sputum?

Patient: A little bit.

Nurse 1: And what color is it?

Patient: Green.

Nurse 1: Green. Have you been running a fever at all with your symptoms?

Patient: I've had a little bit of fever. It's been about 102.

Nurse 1: Okay. Any shortness of breath?

Patient: Uh, it's just kind of hard to breath.

Nurse 1: Okay. Chest pain?

Patient: A little bit.

Nurse 1: Okay. Does anyone in your house smoke?

Patient: No.

Nurse 1: And are you currently a smoker?

Patient: No.

Nurse 1: Have you been exposed to anyone in the last couple weeks that have been sick with flu like symptoms? Pneumonia?

Patient: No.

Nurse 1: Anyone in your family with a history of TB?

Patient: No.

Nurse 1: And have you had a cough greater than 3 weeks?

Patient: It just started about 3 weeks ago.

Nurse 1: Just about 3 weeks ago. And as far as your immunization status, do you receive the pneumonia vaccine at all?

Patient: No.

Nurse 1: Okay. Heather has marked down that you're allergic to penicillin. What side effects do you have with penicillin?

Patient: I get hives.

Nurse 1: Okay. Is there any other medical history? Thyroid?

Patient: No.

Nurse 1: Are you having any pain anywhere at the present time?

Patient: No.

Nurse 1: On the pain scale of zero to ten, you would rate it a zero?

Patient: Probably a one or two, more discomfort.

(Duplicate question—see above)

Nurse 1: Okay. Heather has told me you're allergic to penicillin. What side effects do you notice with the penicillin?

Patient: Hives.

Nurse 1: Hives. Okay. And there's no other medication that you're allergic to?

Patient: No.

Nurse 1: Okay. I'm done my questionnaire here. Heather is going to be doing your vital signs and we'll start that process right now, okay?

Patient: Okay.

Nurse 1: Okay.

Nurse 2: I'm going to take your vital signs. I'm going to lift your bed up to make it a little easier for me. This is a pulse oximeter, it goes on your finger. It will help me determine your heart rate and your level of oxygen in your body. I need to take your blood pressure. I understand sometimes this can be a little uncomfortable. There you go. Will you straighten your arm for me? Thank you. Because of your symptoms that you told Linda I'm going to go ahead and put you on a heart monitor. It will help to make sure your heart is beating at the right rate.

Patient: Okay.

Nurse 2: I will have to expose your chest a little bit for this, is it okay if I expose your chest in front of the people who are in here?

Patient: Yes.

Nurse 2: There you go. Thank you very much.

Nurse 1: Mrs. Jones, one of the things that we need to do is identify the medications that you're currently on. Do you have them with you, or a list?

Patient: My sister has my meds.

Nurse 1: Oh, that is great.

Sister: We brought the bottles because we didn't know if we'd remember everything.

Nurse 1: Okay.

Sister: Here's the cough medicine she's been taking, and the doctor prescribed that about a year ago, I think, for something else, and so she's been using that.

Nurse 1: Okay, so she's been taking that for some recent symptoms and it's prescribed a year ago. Okay.

Sister: Uh huh. And here's her blood pressure medicine.

Nurse 1: Okay. Thank you. That's the Divan. I'll write that down.

Sister: And this doesn't have a label. I think this is her calcium that she's been taking.

Nurse 1: Okay, but we're not too sure, it's not labeled. Okay, I can send that to pharmacy to make sure that we identify that is really calcium.

Sister: Okay, she's also on cholesterol medicine, and I didn't bring that.

Nurse 1: Okay, all right, and we'll call the pharmacy.

Narrator: Notice in this next video clip how the physician collaborates with the patient about care.

■ Confirms the symptoms the patient is having

- Notes the pneumonia protocol has been started
- Performs own focused exam
- Informs the patient regarding the next steps to be taken
- States that the test results confirm pneumonia
- Asks if the patient will agree to being admitted to the hospital
- Reports that she has spoken to her regular physician showing collaboration
- Informs the patient of what unit she will be transferred to
- The physician also asks the patient if she has any further questions
- They physician also reassures the patient by saying, "We will take very good care of you."

Conversation

Doctor: Hi, Miss Jones.

Patient: Hello.

Doctor: I'm Dr. Lynn. I've been here for about 17 years working in the ER so you're in good hands. Tell me how you've been feeling.

Patient: Uh, I've had shortness of breath, cough that I can't get rid of, and a fever.

Doctor: All right. I see the nurses started the pneumonia protocol which we suspect that you have based on your symptoms. So we started an IV and drew some blood, checked your vital signs. You do have a fever. So, all right. Who's your family doctor?

Patient: Dr. Smith.

Doctor: Okay. Well we'll be sure to get a hold of Dr. Smith and let him know what we find. Is it okay if I go ahead and examine you?

Patient: Yes.

Doctor: Take a deep breath. Good. Okay you can lay back. Another deep breath. Okay, you can breathe normal. I'm going to listen to your heart. Okay. I'm going to listen to your stomach. Any nausea or vomiting?

Patient: No.

Doctor: Okay. I'm going to go down and look at your feet for swelling. Doesn't appear to be any swelling. Okay—well we will wait about 15–20 minutes for these test results to come back, and if the test results come back positive for pneumonia then we'll go ahead and start you on IV antibiotic and go from there.

Patient: Okay.

Doctor: All right.

Doctor: Hi, Miss Jones. We got your test results back, and it does confirm that you have pneumonia. Your chest X-ray came back with pneumonia. So if it's okay with you I'd like to admit you, give you some IV antibiotics, which I'm going to ask the nurse to start right now.

Patient: Okay.

Doctor: Give you some Tylenol for your fever. We've gotten a hold of your physician, Dr. Smith and let him know, and he will go ahead and follow up and see you in the hospital.

Patient: Okay.

Doctor: We're going to put you in CCPU (Coronary Care Procedure Unit) which is 3th floor, room 372. It's a private room.

Patient: How long am I going to be here?

Doctor: Dr. Smith will determine that.

Patient: Okay.

Doctor: He'll see you this afternoon or tomorrow. And depending on the progress you're making he'll let you know that.

Patient: Okay.

Doctor: Any other questions?

Patient: I don't think so.

Sister: He'll get all the results that you got down here?

Doctor: Yes. Everything that we've done down here will be communicated. The nurse will report up to the 3rd floor to the nurse up there.

Patient: Okay.

Doctor: Well thank you for coming to Howard.

Patient: Thank you.

Unit Five Comfort and Pain (Video)

Part I Listening & Speaking
Task 1 Listening

Narrator: When we assess symptoms which is subjective information provided by the patient we often use a series of letters, or a mnemonic, to help us remember what to ask.

PQRST:

"P" stands for "Provoke". What causes or makes the symptom worse?

"Q" stands for "Quality". Encourage the patient to use their own words to describe their condition.

"R" stands for "Radiation". If pain is involved, does the pain radiate to a different part of the body?

"S" stands for "Severity". Have the patient use a scale to rate the severity of their shortness of breath.

You could have the patient say a sentence and you could count the number of words the patient can say without stopping. If the patient's condition worsens he or she may be able to say fewer words without stopping to take a breath. If the patient is having pain, a scale of 0 to 10 can be used. Zero indicates no pain, and 10 indicates the most severe pain.

"T" stands for triggering factors. When and how long has the patient had shortness of breath or pain?

Another mnemonic you might use is: WILDA, W   I   L   D   A

Words—Patient's statement about the symptom.

Intensity—Use a scale like the 0 to 10 pain intensity scale, or the Visual Analog Scale (VAS), or the extent to which the symptom is interfering with the patient's functioning (0 indicates no pain, and 10 indicates intense, incapacitating pain). The patient should also be asked what makes their pain better or worse.

Location—"where is your pain?" or "Do you have pain in more than one area?"

Duration—Pain may be constant or intermittent. Asking the patient, "How long does the pain last?" and/or "Is the pain always there, or does it come and go?" or "How much time do you have in between periods of pain?"

Aggravating and alleviating factors - Asking the patient to describe what factors aggravate or alleviate their pain will help in planning the interventions. A typical question might be, "What makes the pain better or worse? " Are there any associated symptoms such as nausea, vomiting, constipation, sleepiness, and weakness?

As you watch this next video watch for the nurse to ask these questions and how the nurse offers to help the patient with pain relief.

Conversation

Nurse: Good morning, Mrs. Smith. How are you?

Patient: Good.

Nurse: My name is Heather and I'm going to be your nurse today. How are you feeling?

Patient: Pretty good.

Nurse: Are you having any pain?

Patient: Yes, I am having a little bit of pain.

Nurse: Where is it at?

Patient: Um, underneath my knee.

Nurse: Right here under your knee?

Patient: Yes. Coming up toward my thigh a little.

Nurse: Okay. That's probably some incisional pain. Could you describe it for me?

Patient: Um, it just feels like it's pulling a lot.

Nurse: Okay, is it a constant pain or more of an intermittent pain?

Patient: It's constant.

Nurse: On a scale of 1 to 10, how would you rate it?

Patient: Uh, probably a 7.

Nurse: Okay. Well I can do a couple of things for you. We can reposition you if you want. We can see if that would work.

Patient: Okay.

Nurse: Okay, I'm just going to kind of move your leg here. The pain on the back of your leg is probably from the surgery itself when they did the manipulation of your knee. That can be rather painful and it causes a lot of inflammation.

Patient: Okay.

Nurse: So what I'm going to do is go get you some Toradol. It's an antiinflammatory, and that's going to help you with your pain. As soon as you're done with therapy we'll unclamp your block and then we'll be able to get some more of that numbing medication into your femoral nerve, that's going to help a lot too.

Patient: Okay.

Nurse: Is there anything else I can do for you?

Patient: No, I think that's all.

Nurse: All right. I'm going to be right back, okay?

Patient: Okay. Thank you.

Nurse: Thank you.

Unit Six Medication Administration (Video)

Part I Listening & Speaking
Task 1 Listening

Nurse: Well hello, Tammy. I guess you're going to stay in the hospital with us.

Patient: Yes.

Nurse: I'm so sorry to hear that you've got pneumonia, but you're in the best place. We'll take very good care of you. We've got a room on the 3rd floor.

Patient: Okay.

Nurse: You'll be going up momentarily, just as soon as we get your antibiotic started, okay? We have a very safe way of checking medications to the right patient so what I'm going to do is scan your bracelet that identifies you, and also I'm going to scan the medication that's been ordered by the physician.

Patient: Okay.

Nurse: So if you could tell me your name and birth date.

Patient: Tammy Jones, 10-2-63.

Nurse: Okay. I'm going to scan the medication now.

Patient: Okay.

Nurse: This is your Tylenol. I'm going to scan your bracelet again.

Sister: And what does Tylenol do?

Nurse: It's for her fever.

Sister: Okay.

Nurse: Okay. Now I'm going to scan the medication. Your fever was 102.2 so we need to get that under control. So here's your Tylenol and your water.

Patient: And this is my Tylenol?

Nurse: This is your Tylenol. Here you go ma'am. Okay—all right, we're going to get that antibiotic started right now.

Sister: Will that antibiotic hurt when it's going in?

Nurse: No, this antibiotic should not hurt while it's infusing. At any time should your arm get sensitive from the antibiotic, or you start to develop pain, please let us know because that should not happen.

Patient: Okay.

Nurse: Okay. I'm just going to hook up your IV right now, Tammy. I'll get this going right now. At any time that it starts to feel uncomfortable, you have any pain that's unusual, we want you to let us know.

Patient: Okay.

Nurse: Okay. This is on a pump and it will infuse at the correct rate at the correct amount. Is there anything else I can do for you right now, Tammy?

Patient: I don't think so.

Nurse: Okay.

Patient: How long before I get up to a room?

Nurse: I'm just going to call the nurse on your floor right now. She should be ready for report and we'll get you upstairs just as soon as she takes report. And we should get you up there momentarily.

Patient: Okay.

Nurse: All right. Well I hope you get to feeling better soon. So thank you for choosing Howard, and we'll get that done right now, okay?

Patient: Okay, thank you.

Unit Seven Specimen Collection (Video)

Part I Listening & Speaking
Task 1 Listening

In this clip please note how the nurse explains to the patient about the diagnostic studies to be performed, including a chest X-ray and blood work.

The nurse washes her hands, puts on gloves and makes sure the equipment is ready. She indicates that she will leave the "straw" in the patient's arm to give medications through if needed.

After the blood draw the nurse then tells the patient how long it will take to get the results and then thanks the patient. Listen to how the nurse uses everyday words, instead of medical terms including words like straw for IV cannula, or rubber band for tourniquet and salt water for normal saline.

Nurse 1: Mrs. Jones, I've noticed that your oxygen level is 92%. That's a little bit on the low side. We have some protocols for I think that you might have pneumonia and we have some protocols, that we do follow the emergency department. So how this will be going to come in? And she's going to place you on some oxygen therapy. First, sneeze pump will go in your nose and help you feel a lot better. Also we are going to be drawing some blood through an IV and the doctor likes to have a chest X-ray done that we follow through on those protocols. We will be getting that done momentarily. Is that OK with you?

Patient: OK.

Nurse 1: OK. Thank you.

Nurse 2: When I'm back I'm going to wash my hands and set my equipment for the blood-draw and put you on some oxygen, OK? Tell me your name and date birth again.

Patient: Tammy Jones. 10.2. 63.

Nurse 2: Can I see your wrist-let? Thank you. All right. What I'm going to do is leave a little straw in when I get the blood that way we need to give any medication later. We don't have to poke you again.

Patient: OK.

Nurse 2: The very first thing I'm going to do is just to look for a vein. It is a little rubber band. I will tie it around your arm. It's going to be a little uncomfortable. It looks like I've found a good vein right here. I'm going to undo the rubber band. You can go to have a relaxation on your arm and I'm going to clean the site. Just cold them right now. We will let that dry. And I'm going to get everything else ready. All right. That looks to be dry. I'm going to tie the rubber band again.

Patient: Can my sister come up so that I can squeeze her hands?

Nurse 2: Absolutely.

Patient's sister: It's going to be all right.

Nurse 2: The poke will be overshot and that will be just a straw. All right. Big poke. Good, the needle's gone. Now I'm going to draw some blood from that site. Good. Make grail dry one more two.

Patient: Are you almost done?

Nurse 2: I'm almost done and I'm going to tap this. I'm going to loosen the rubber band. OK. Now I'm just putting on some tubing that has some water in it that will keep the IV flowing well. Can you feel, you might feel a little cold this in your arm. I'm just flushing. Hard parts are all over. The elastic band will tell the date of time. I'm just going to tape this. This straw does band. It's not a needle in your arm. It might be felt odd when you band but it won't hurt. So feel free of it. Be comfortable. I'm going to label this blood.

Patient's sister: How soon will we have these results back?

Nurse 2: After the doctor orders the tests. It will be 2 hours and 45 minutes before the results come back. Our doctor will then come in and tell you what those results are and if we need to do anything further.

Patient's sister: OK.

Nurse 2: Let me step back a moment and put some alcohol on my hands. I'm going to put you on some oxygen. Have you worn oxygen before?

Patient: No.

Nurse 2: It's going to tickle a little bit. Some people say it smells a little. It's right in your nose and around your ears. Is that comfortable?

Patient: Yes.

Nurse 2: OK. I'm all done. Is there anything else I can do for you?

Patient: I don't think so.

Nurse 2: Thank you very much for your help.

Patient: Thank you.

Nurse 2: I'm all done. Here's your call if you need anything. Is there anything else I can do for you?

Patient: I don't think so. Thank you very much.

Nurse 2: Thank you very much.

Nurse 1: Hi, Mrs Jones.

Patient: Hi.

Nurse 1: Hi, I'm just going to review some, a few things with Hector. I've spoken to doctor Lam about you. And she's going to be in momentarily.

Nurse 2: As we discussed about the pneumonia, sorry pneumonia protocols. She had a fever about 102. So I've drawn some blood and she's on oxygen. And she's all yours.

Nurse 1: OK. Thank you.

Nurse 2: Thank you.

Nurse 1: With the pneumonia protocols, the next step, Mrs. Jones, will be a bedside chest X-ray. We will ask your sister to stay outside just she doesn't have exposure. We will get that done. We will get your label to the lab with your oxygen on. It really looks like you're improving greatly. It's 96%. I'm really, really happy with that. Is there anything else I can do for you when you are waiting for doctor Lam to come in?

Patient: Not right now.

Patient's sister: Do you know how long is it going to be before the doctor gets here?

Nurse 1: It's going to about 10 minutes. The X-ray is ready to command and take your bedside chest X-ray. And then the doctor will be in to see you.

Patient: OK.

Nurse 1: Are you having any change in your pain, level, or any change in your symptoms since you've been here?

Patient: No. Just the oxygen makes me feel a little better.

Nurse 1: OK. If there is anything we can do for you or any change in your symptoms for your hair, we want to make sure you usually call.

Patient's sister: Can she have something to drink?

Nurse 1: Yes. We can get that for you right away, ma'am.

Patient's sister: OK. All right. That will be good.

Unit Eight Care of Surgical Clients (Video)

Part I Listening & Speaking
Task 1 Listening

Narrator: Identify the errors the nurse makes in caring for the patient in the following clip.

VIDEO (IMPROPER EXAMPLE)

Nurse: All right. So here's your consent form for the surgery.

Patient: Oh, okay.

Nurse: You know what you're having done, right?

Patient: Uh, yes.

Nurse: Did the doctor explain anything?

Patient: Well, not really.

Nurse: Okay so~

Patient: I did have a few questions.

Nurse: Well you're going to have to go and ask them when you get downstairs because he should have done that before, you know, today. So~

Patient: Oh, well my family's not here yet, and I haven't told them yet even.

Nurse: Well you probably should have told them yesterday because you knew we were going to do this this morning, and they're running a really tight schedule downstairs, so we're going to have to get you down there. They're here to take you down right now.

Patient: Oh, okay.

Nurse: So I'm going to have to have you sign this for me real quick.

Patient: Okay.

Transport: Excuse me, I've got to unplug her bed.

Nurse: All right.

Patient: Okay.

Nurse: All right, well see you later.

Patient: Bye.

Transport: Well, we're taking you to surgery.

Patient: Okay.

Transport: So, hope you're ready. Here we go.

Patient: I guess I am.

Narrator: What does the nurse do better this time?

VIDEO (PROPER EXAMPLE)

Nurse: Good morning, Mrs. Smith.

Patient: Good morning.

Nurse: How are you?

Patient: Okay.

Nurse: All right. I see you're going to have a knee replacement today.

Patient: Yes.

Nurse: Do you feel like the doctor explained that procedure to you? Are there any questions that you can think of?

Patient: Well, I just don't know what to expect.

Nurse: Okay. Well here, you went through the joint replacement class for our hospital, correct?

Patient: Yes.

Nurse: Okay, well I brought the book in and this just has a little bit of information about it. And we can kind of go through that if you'd like.

Patient: Okay.

Nurse: Okay, I'm going to give that to you. Basically what's going to happen is they're going to take you downstairs. They'll take you on your bed, and you will come back on your bed, okay?

Patient: Okay, okay.

Nurse: Your family can go down with you, and we have a waiting room for them. When you're done with your surgery, the doctor's going to come out and speak with them, and he'll update them on how you're doing. It's going to be a little bit cold down there, and the lights are going to be a little bright. Sometimes that can be a little frightening but there will be plenty of people in there with you to help you out.

Patient: Okay.

Nurse: We're going to have to put a catheter in keep your bladder drained during the surgery, and that will stay in for two days. When we bring you back up here you'll also have a pain block in your knee, and that's going to help numb that leg up for the next couple of days to alleviate the pain, okay?

Patient: Okay.

Nurse: You'll have an incision along the front of your knee. It'll be about 4 to 5 inches in length and they'll have staples in there. They're titanium staples and they are waterproof, and we'll have that wrapped up and dressed up so that you don't have to look at that until you're ready. Do you have any other questions for me?

Patient: No, I think you covered it all. Thank you.

Nurse: Okay. Well I'm going to show you this is your consent form. Are you allergic to anything?

Patient: No, not that I know of.

Nurse: Okay, and you're going to have a right total knee arthroplasty, and I'm going to give you an opportunity to read through this consent form, and then you can let me know if you have any questions, okay?

Patient: Okay.

Nurse: So I'm going to give that to you here.

Patient: All right, thank you.

Nurse: You're very welcome. I think we're done. Is there anything else I can do for you?

Patient: No.

Nurse: Okay, well thank you so much, and they'll be up to get you shortly.

Patient: All right.

Nurse: You take care down there and we'll see you when you get back.

Patient: All right.

Nurse: Thank you.

Transport 1: Hi, I'm Jane and this is Laura. We're going to take you down.

Transport 2: Hi.

Transport 1: Can you tell us your name and date of birth?

Patient: Hello. Mrs. Smith, 10-15-82.

Transport 1: Okay. We're going to take you downstairs for your surgery.

Transport 2: We'll try to be real careful with your bed and not bump you into anything, but make sure you keep your hands and feet inside, and don't put them up on the sides, okay?

Patient: Okay.

Transport 2: Here we go.

Unit Nine Emergency Nursing (Video)

Part I Listening & Speaking
Task 1 Listening

In this video clip the patient is complaining of shortness of breath. Please watch as the nurse answers the call light, assesses the patient's signs and symptoms and offers reassurance.

Listen for the questions the nurse is asking the patient. Notice how the nurse calls for more help when she realizes the patient is having trouble breathing.

　　We call this a rapid response. The purpose is to catch the patient's condition before it worsens so the patient does not have to go to an intensive care unit.

Nurse: Your call light's on.

Patient: I just feel really short of breath. I haven't been able to catch my breath.

Nurse: Yeah, you look you're having some trouble breathing. You know what, I'm going to go ahead and start getting your vital signs and then I'm going to call for some help. How long has this been going on?

Patient: About a minute or so.

Nurse: Just a minute or so. Well all right. I want you to try and stay calm and take some deep and slow breaths. I'm going to just ask for some help and I'll be right back. Could somebody please call a rapid response? I don't want to leave my patient; she's not doing very well.

Nurse 2: What's going on?

Nurse: Hi, I'm glad you guys are here. Mrs. Smith has started having some recent trouble breathing. She came in for a DVT (deep vein thrombosis). I went ahead and started getting her vital signs. Her sats (oxygen saturation) are only 84%, and she's really having trouble catching her breath.

Nurse 2: Okay. Why don't we try to get some oxygen on her?

Nurse: I heard some crackles in her lungs about an hour ago when I listened. They weren't very bad, I did notify the doctor, but he didn't order anything at that time.

Nurse 3: Okay. Who is her doctor?

Nurse: Dr. Jones. And in the past when she's has crackles he's ordered some Lasix. I think that might be helpful to her.

Nurse 3: I would say let's get 20 of Lasix and order a stat chest x-ray, and go ahead and get that up. (Note: Some American hospitals have protocols, like starting oxygen therapy and giving certain medications, nurses can begin while waiting for a physician for patients in emergency situations). And I'll go ahead and get her blood pressure and stuff, while you're getting that.

Nurse: Okay. What I heard you say is to order a stat chest x-ray and get 20 milligrams of IV Lasix. (Repeating orders enhances communication and decreased the likelihood of errors).

Nurse 3: Yes. Thank you, Laura.

Nurse: Okay, I'll be right back with those.

Nurse 2: All right, do we have a fresh set of vital signs?

Nurse 3: Yes.

Narrator: For more information about rapid response teams please view the link below: http: //www.aarc.org/resources/rapid_response/. Did you hear the way the first nurse told the others on the team about the patient's condition? Sometimes we use something called an SBAR. An SBAR stands for:

Situation—What is happening right now with the patient? Background—What in the patient's history is relevant to the current situation?

Assessment—What are the patient's vital signs, signs and symptoms?

Recommendation—What does the nurse believe will help the patient at this time?

If an order is given by a physician the nurse must repeat it back to avoid error. Now listen to the video clip again and listen the portions of the SBAR.

Unit Ten Family Visit (Audio)

Part I Listening & Speaking
Task 1 Listening

Interview Bridget Levich, a diabetes resource nurse for UC Davis Medical Center's Home Care Department. She is one of many registered nurses who visit patients in their homes.

Q: What's a diabetes resource nurse?

A: I specialize in diabetes, so most of my patients are learning how to live with this chronic disease.

Q: Why did you choose this specialty?

A: Early in my nursing career, I actually was diagnosed with type I diabetes. I really appreciate the need for patients with diabetes to be self-managing and learn how to be in charge of their own illness. So, I teach patients not only as a nurse but as someone who's living with the disease as well.

Q: Why do you think patients need home care?

A: The patients are getting discharged from the hospital much sicker. Patients come home with lots of skilled needs that are very difficult for the patient without education or without a skilled person to deliver them.

Q: You have been a hospital nurse. Why did you change to be a home care nurse?

A: I discovered that working in a hospital didn't allow me enough time to teach my patients how to "manage" their illnesses. So after going back to school and earning my public health certificate, I landed in the home health department.

Q: Do you find patients like home care more than hospital care?

A: Certainly. When I work in a patient's home, it means that I am able to check a patient's vitals, as well as teach them how to take care of their own illness in the comfort of the patient's living room.

Q: Besides the nurse, are there other medical staff working in the home health department? How do you collaborate with them?

A: Often, after making initial contact with a patient and assessing his or her home, I may call on other skilled professionals to help. I collaborate with the patient's physician on each case, but it's the day-to-day autonomy that I enjoy.

Unit Eleven Community Health Nursing (Audio)

Part I Listening & Speaking
Task 1 Listening
A conversation

T: What is Alzheimer's disease?

S: Alzheimer's disease is a brain disease that slowly destroys memory and thinking skills and, eventually, the ability to carry out the simplest tasks.

T: What is typically the first sign of Alzheimer's disease?

S: Memory problems are typically one of the first signs of Alzheimer's disease, though different people may have different initial symptoms. A decline in other aspects of thinking, such as finding the right words, vision/spatial issues, and impaired reasoning or judgment, may also signal the very early stages of Alzheimer's disease.

T: What are the causes of Alzheimer's disease?

S: So far as I know, the causes of Alzheimer's disease remain a mystery. Some studies suggest that one or more factors other than heredity may determine whether people develop the disease; some researchers suspect that health problems such as hypertension, atherosclerosis, high cholesterol levels, or other cardiovascular problems may play a role in the development of the disease.

T: What are the stages in the development of Alzheimer's disease?

S: People with Alzheimer's exhibit different symptoms as the disease progresses, but most symptoms are either cognitive or behavioral. The symptoms of Alzheimer's can also be collapsed into three broad stages: early, middle, and late. In early-stage Alzheimer's, individuals may still function quite well overall. Although they may be aware of the increasing difficulty with certain tasks, they are also often quite skilled at hiding this from others by deflecting questions, changing the topic, or relying on their family or loved ones to make decisions or answer questions. Moderate, or mid-stage, Alzheimer's is often the most difficult stage. While some individuals remain "pleasantly confused" throughout the entire disease, many display inappropriate behaviors and emotions.In the final stage of Alzheimer's, people are often are quite immobile, and spend much of their time in bed or in a wheelchair.

T: How could Alzheimer's disease be prevented?

S: Currently, no medicines or other treatments are known to prevent Alzheimer's disease, but scientists are studying many possibilities. These possibilities include lifestyle factors such as exercise and physical activity, a healthy diet, and mentally stimulating activities. In addition to lifestyle factors, scientists have found clues that some long-term health conditions, like heart disease, high blood pressure, and diabetes, are related to Alzheimer's disease. It's possible that controlling these conditions will reduce the risk of developing Alzheimer's.

Unit Twelve Caring for Terminally ill Patients (Audio)

Part I Listening & Speaking
Task 1 Listening

Hospice Helps Patients Live Their Final Days

Welcome to American Mosaicfrom VOA Learning English. I'm June Simms.

When people hear the word hospice, they usually link it to death and dying. But as Marsha James tells us, hospice is focused more about providing care, comfort and support to patients during their final days of life.

Faye and Wayne Payne lived a rich and interesting life before settling down in rural Virginia. But their peaceful existence was crushed when they learned that Faye had lung cancer.

The 70-year-old retiredsecretary went through a series of aggressive medical treatments that left her weak and underweight.

"I did the radiation, and I did the chemo, and after I had the last scan done they realized I had more cancer coming up here. And I said 'no more.'"

Faye decided to seek hospice care after talking about the future with her family and doctors. Social worker Robin Johnson is part of the hospice team that visits Faye in her home.

"The nurse is looking at the medical things and the social worker at the psycho-social spiritual things, which can encompass a lot."

Faye Payne explains the value of her hospice care.

"They helped me realize that, yes, death is coming. And they've helped me get ready. I now have everything lined up and ready to go."

Hospice care helps for family members too, like Faye's husband.

"They come along and they take her blood pressure and check her hearing and get her medication and it's made life a whole lot easier for both of us."

Melissa Mills is assistant director of patient services at Hospice of the Rapidan.

The organization serves terminally ill patients in several counties in the state of Virginia.

"We're all here for the same mission and that's to help our patients die with compassion and dignity."

Seventy-four-year-old Jim Sykes learned that he had head and neck cancer two years ago. He has been receiving hospice care at home for seven months.

"I would advise anybody that needs help like this extra support, that hospice is what they need"

Lisa Stone is Jim's social worker.

"A lot of my visits are providing a lot of supportive listening. Jim has his black book of photos so we do what I like to call photo therapy."

Eric Lindner has been a hospice volunteer since 2009 and has written about his experiences. He believes hospice provides a support system that is largely missing in American culture.

"I've travelled a fair bit—China, Africa, other places—and the elders are embraced and taken into the family. In this country just the way it's developed, maybe that's the role that hospice has tried to fill a little bit."

That support has helped patients like Faye Payne enjoy her quality of life today. And she says when the time comes for her to leave this earth, she is ready.

"I was born on July 16th, 1942, but my dad was working on the railroad and he died April 16th, 1942, so I want to get to see my dad one day, that's the main thing. I have no regrets and I'm not afraid."

Unit Thirteen Rehabilitation Nursing

Part I Listening & Speaking
Task 1 Listening

A stroke, sometimes called a "brain attack," occurs when blood flow to the brain is interrupted. When a stroke occurs, brain cells in the immediate area begin to die because they stop getting the oxygen and nutrients they need to function.

Although stroke is a disease of the brain, it can affect the entire body. The effects of a stroke range from mild to severe and can include paralysis, problems with thinking, problems with speaking, and emotional problems. Patients may also experience pain or numbness after a stroke. Because stroke injures the brain, people may not realize that they are having a stroke. To a bystander, someone having a stroke may just look unaware or confused. Stroke victims have the best chance if someone around them recognizes the symptoms and acts quickly.

The symptoms of stroke are distinct because they happen quickly:

- Sudden numbness or weakness of the face, arm, or leg (especially on one side of the body)
- Sudden confusion, trouble speaking or understanding speech
- Sudden trouble seeing in one or both eyes
- Sudden trouble walking, dizziness, loss of balance or coordination
- Sudden severe headache with no known cause

Stroke is a medical emergency. Every minute counts when someone is having a stroke. The longer blood flow is cut off to the brain, the greater the damage. Immediate treatment can save people's lives and enhance their chances for successful recovery.

The best treatment for stroke is prevention. There are several risk factors that increase your chances of having a stroke:

- High blood pressure
- Heart disease
- Smoking
- Diabetes
- High cholesterol

If you smoke, quit. If you have high blood pressure, heart disease, diabetes, or high cholesterol, getting them under control and keeping them under control, will greatly reduce your chances of having a stroke.

Unit Fourteen Traditional Chinese Medicine

Part I Listening & Speaking
Task 1 Listening

Food As Medicine

Food acts as medicine, to maintain, prevent, and treat disease. The nutrients in food enable the cells in our bodies to perform their necessary functions. Nutrients are the nourishing substances in food that are essential for the growth, development and maintenance of body functions. The food we eat gives our bodies the "information" and materials they need to function properly. If we don't get the right information, our metabolic processes suffer and our health declines. In short, what we eat is central to our health.

The following are some suggestions on how to take food as medicine in our daily life.

1. Eat a variety of foods. Studies show that people who eat a variety of foods are healthier, live longer, and have a reduced risk of diseases, such as heart disease, cancer, and diabetes. Food variety means including foods such as fruit, vegetables, meat, fish, and dairy products. By eating a diet that includes a variety of foods, you will be providing the nutrients that the body needs.

2. Increase fruits and vegetables. Fruits and vegetables are not only full of vitamins and minerals, but they contain beneficial plant nutrients to defend the body against disease, radiation, weather, insects, and anything that may threaten its survival. When we eat these plants, we also benefit from the protection of the plant nutrients.

3. Choose whole grains. Fiber in whole grains makes us feel full faster and longer; therefore, it may prevent overeating. Fiber also plays an important role in the digestive system, allowing nutrients to be more fully absorbed and slowing the rise in blood sugar glucose, as well as aiding in the elimination of waste.

4. Drink water. Water is needed for the digestion, absorption, and transportation of nutrients. Water keeps skin smooth and soft, reduces toxicity, and flushes toxins and excess salt from the body. It also regulates body temperature and is useful in managing hunger. Note that as you get older, your thirst sense is diminished. It is especially important for older adults to drink water before they become thirsty.

5. Include green tea. Numerous studies have shown an association between the consumption of green tea and protection against cancer. Green tea and its extracts have also been used for improving mental alertness, aiding in weight loss, protecting skin from sun damage, and lowering cholesterol. The green tea also increases fat burning, as well as improving insulin sensitivity and glucose control during moderate exercise.

6. Avoid overeating. Pay attention to what, when, and why you eat. Keeping a food diary helps people lose weight. Try to avoid eating standing up, watching TV, or driving. Eat slowly and chew. You will get more "food experience" from fewer calories. Eat smaller, more frequent meals (every three to four hours). Skipping meals causes excessive hunger and may lead to eating larger portions at the next meal.

7. Limit processed foods. On the one hand, processed foods lack nutrients. On the other hand, they often contain artificial color, additives, flavorings, and chemically altered fats and sweeteners. While some of these processed foods claim to be low in fat, they are often high in sugar. A common recommendation for healthy eating is to shop around the part of the supermarket where the fresh, natural, non-processed foods tend to be.

Common Medical Word Roots & Affixes

汉语 / 英语常用词根例

颜色系统

色 color

chrom(o) monochrome 单色；achromatopsia 全色盲

红 red

rub bilirubinuria 胆红素尿

erythro erythrocin 红霉素；erythrocyte 红细胞

黄 yellow

lute(o) lutein 叶黄素；luteosterone 黄体酮

flav(o) flavacin 黄曲霉素

绿 green

chlor(o) chlorophyll 叶绿素

verd(o) verdoglobinuria 胆绿蛋白尿

蓝 blue

cyant(o) cyanein 蓝菌素；cyanosis 发绀；青紫

紫 purple

purp purpura 紫癜

violet ultraviolet 紫外线

viol violamine 紫胺

白 white

leuc(o) leucocyte 白细胞

leuk(o) leukemia 白血病

albi albinism 白化病

灰白 gray

grise(o) grisein 灰霉素

poli(o) poliosis 白发症；poliomyelitis 脊髓灰质炎

黑 black

mela melasma 黑斑病

melan(o)　melanin 黑色素；melanoma 黑色素瘤；melanocyte 黑素细胞

方位系统
上 up

epi　epicytoma 上皮瘤

super　superconductor 超导体；

supra　supracapsulin (adrenalin, epinephrine) 肾上腺素

下 down

infer(o)　inferolateral 下外侧的

infra　infraorbital 眶下的

sub　subaxillary 腋下的

hypo　hypodermic 皮下的

左 left

leva　levamizole 左旋咪唑

levo　levocardiogram 左侧心电图

右 right

dextr(o)　dextrocardiogram 右侧心电图

dexter　dextrocular 惯用右眼的

前 front

ante　proantecubital 肘前的

pre　preoperative 术前的；prostatic 前列腺的；prophylaxis 预防法

后 behind

post　postpartum 产后的

retr(o)　retrobulbar 眼球后的

内 inside

endo　intraendocardium 心内膜；endocrine 内分泌的

中心 center

centro　centrocyte 中央细胞；centrokinesis 中枢性运动

中间 middle

medi(o)　media 介质；血管中层；mediocidin 中霉素

外 outside

ect(o)　ectohormone 外激素

exo　exocervix 外子宫颈

extra　extracorporeal 体外的；extracranial 颅外的

周围 around

circum　circumcision 包皮环切术

peri　periodontitis 牙周炎

呼吸系统
呼吸 breath

pnea　tachypnea 呼吸过速；bradypnea 呼吸过缓

pneum(o)　dyspnea 呼吸困难；pneumothorax 气胸

spir(o)　expiration 呼气；inspiration 吸气

鼻 nose

rhin(o)　rhinitis 鼻炎；rhinorrhoea 鼻漏

喉 larynx

laryng(o)　laryngitis 喉炎；laryngectomy 喉切除术

气管 windpipe

trache(o)　tracheotomy 气管切开术；tracheobronchitis 气管支气管炎

支气管 bronchi

bronch(o)　bronchiectasis 支气管扩张；bronchitis 支气管炎

肺 lung

pneumon(o)　pneumonia 肺炎；bronchopneumonia 支气管肺炎

pulmo(n)　pulmonary 肺的；bronchopulmonary 支气管肺的

胸膜 pleura

pleur(o)　pleuritis 胸膜炎；pleural 胸膜的

循环系统

心 heart

cardi(o)　electrocardiogram 心电图；phonocardiogram 心音图

瓣膜 valve

valvul(o)　valvulitis 瓣膜炎；multivalvular 多瓣膜的

血管 vessel

vas(o)　vasculitis 血管炎；vasopressin 血管升压素

angi(o)　angiotensin 血管紧张素；angiography 血管造影

动脉 artery

arteri(o)　arteriography 动脉造影术；arteritis 动脉炎；endoarteritis 动脉内膜炎

静脉 vein

ven(o)　venous 静脉的；intravenous 内静脉的

phleb(o)　phlebitis 静脉炎；phlebography 静脉造影

脉搏 pulse

puls(o)　pulseless 无脉的；pulsed 脉冲的

消化系统

咽 pharynx

pharyng(o)　pharyngitis 咽炎；craniopharyngioma 颅咽管瘤

食管 esophagus

esophag(o)　esophagoscope 食管镜；gastroesophageal 胃食管的

胃 stomach

gastr(o)　gastritis 胃炎；gastroscopy 胃镜检查；gastropathy 胃病

stomach(o)　stomachache 胃痛

肠 **intestine**

enter(o)　enteritis 肠炎；enterovirus 肠道病毒

十二指肠 **duodenum**

duoden(o)　duodenal 十二指肠的；gastroduodenal 胃十二指肠

结肠 **colon**

col(o)　colon(o)　colonoscopy 结肠镜检查；colitis 结肠炎

消化 **digestion**

peps(o)　dyspepsia 消化不良；pepsin 胃蛋白酶

gest(o)　digestive 消化的；digestible 可消化的

直肠 **rectum**

rect(o)　rectocele 直肠膨出；rectouterine 直肠子宫

procto　proctoptosis 直肠脱垂；proctoscopy 直肠镜检查

胆囊 **gallbladder; cholecyst**

cholecyst(o)　cholecystitis 胆囊炎；cholecystolithiasis/ cholelithiasis 胆囊结石病（或胆石症）

肝 **liver**

hepat(o)　hepatitis 肝炎；hepatorrhexis 肝破裂

胆管 **bile duct**

cholangi(o)　cholangitis 胆管炎；cholangiography 胆管造影术

阑尾 **appendix**

appendic(o)　appendicitis 阑尾炎；appendicectomy 阑尾切除术

泌尿系统

尿 **urine**

urin(o)　urinary 尿的；urinogenital 泌尿生殖的

ur(o)　hematuria 血尿；polyuria 多尿症

肾 **kidney**

ren(o)　suprarenal 肾上的；renovascular 肾血管的

nephr(o)　nephritis 肾炎；hydronephrosis 肾积水

膀胱 **bladder**

vesic(o)　vesical 膀胱的；rectovesical 直肠膀胱的

cyst(o)　cystitis 膀胱炎；cystostomy 膀胱造瘘术

尿道 **urethra**

urethr(o)　urethritis 尿道炎；urethroscopy 尿道镜检查

meat(o)　meatotomy 尿道口切开术；meatorrhaphy 尿道口缝术

睾丸 **testis**

test(o)　testosterone 睾酮

testicul(o)　testicular 睾丸的

orchi(o)　orchitis 睾丸炎

didym(o)　epididymis 附睾

前列腺 **prostate**

prostat(o)   prostatic 前列腺的；prostatitis 前列腺炎

肾盂 **renal pelvis**

pelvi(o)   pelvioplasty 肾盂造影术

pyel(o)   pyelonephritis 肾盂肾炎；pyelography 肾盂造影术

生殖系统

生殖 **reproduction**

genit(o)   genital 生殖的；urogenital 泌尿生殖的

子宫 **womb**

uter(o)   uterine 子宫的；extrauterine 子宫外的

hyster(o)   hysterotomy 子宫切开术

metr(o)   perimetrium 子宫外膜

膀胱 **bladder**

vesic(o)   vesical 膀胱的；rectovesical 直肠膀胱的

cyst(o)   cystitis 膀胱炎；cystostomy 膀胱造瘘术

阴道 **vagina**

vagin(o)   vaginitis 阴道炎

colp(o)   colposcopy 阴道镜检查；colpoperineoplasty 阴道会阴成形术

月经 **menstruation**

men(o)   menopause 绝经；amenorrhea 闭经

胚胎 **embryo**

embry(o)   embryology 胚胎学；tubalembryo 胚胎输卵管

羊膜，羊水 **amnion**

amni(o)   amniotic 羊膜的；amniocentesis 羊膜穿刺术；amnioscopy 羊膜镜检查

胎盘 **placenta**

placent(o)   placental 胎盘的；uteroplacental 子宫胎盘的

胎儿 **fetus**

fet(o)   fetal 胎儿的；fetocardiogram 胎儿心动图

产次 **parity**

para   primipara 初产妇；multipara 多产妇

卵泡 **follicle**

follicul(o)   follicular 卵泡的；folliculosis 卵泡增殖

卵巢 **ovary**

ovari(o)   ovariotomy 卵巢切除术；ovariotubal 卵巢输卵管的

精子 **semen**

semin(o)   seminal 精液的；insemination 受精

阴囊 **scrotum**

scrot(o)   scrotitis 阴囊炎；scrotectomy 阴囊切除术

阴茎 **penis**

penis phall(o) penitis 阴茎炎；phallalgia 阴茎痛

内分泌系统
分泌 secretion
crin(o) endocrine 内分泌
secret(o) secretive 分泌的
腺 gland
aden(o) adenoma 腺瘤；adenomyosis 子宫腺肌病
垂体 pituitary
pitui pituitary 垂体；hypopituitarism 垂体功能减退；pituicyte 垂体细胞
hypophys hypophyseal 垂体的
甲状腺 thyroid
thyr(o) thyroiditis 甲状腺炎；thyroxine 甲状腺素；thyrotrophin 促甲状腺激素
肾上腺 adrenal
adren(o) adrenalitis 肾上腺炎；adrenaline 肾上腺素
胸腺 thymus
thym(o) thymosin 胸腺素；thymoma 胸腺瘤
葡萄糖 glucose
gluc(o) glucagon 胰高血糖素；glucokinase 葡萄糖激酶
钙 calcium
calc(i) calcification 钙化；cholecalciferol 胆钙化醇

神经系统
脑 brain
encephal(o) encephalitis 脑炎；encephalopathy 脑病；encephalomyelitis 脑脊髓炎
大脑 cerebrum
crecbr(o) crecbral 大脑的；crecbrovascular 脑血管的
小脑 cerebellum
cerebell(o) archicerebellum 原小脑；cerebrocerebellum 皮层小脑
丘脑 thalamus
thalam(o) metathalamus 后丘脑；epithalamus 上丘脑
髓质 marrow
medull(o) medullary 髓质的；adrenomedullin 肾上腺髓质素
脑膜，脊膜 membrane
mening(o) meningitis 脑膜炎；leptomeningitis 软脑膜炎；pachymeningitis 硬脑膜炎
脊柱 spine
spin(o) spinocerebellum 脊柱小脑；cerebrospinal 脑脊的
精神，意志 mind
psych(o) psychopathology 精神病理学；psychostimulant 精神兴奋剂
神经 nerve

neur(o)   neurology 神经病学；neurotmesis 神经断伤

蛛网膜 arachnoid

arachn (o)   arachnoidal 蛛网膜的；arachnoiditis 蛛网膜炎；subarachnoid 蛛网膜下

狂，癖 madness

mania(c)   erotomania 色情狂；tocomania 产后躁狂；dipsomania 酒狂

皮肤与感觉系统

眼 eye

ocul(o)   electrooculogram 眼电图

ophthalm(o)   ophthalmopathy 眼病

角膜 cornea

kerat(o)   keratitis 角膜炎；keratomalacia 角膜软化症

结膜 conjunctiva

conjunctiv(o)   conjunctival 结膜的；conjunctivtis 结膜炎；keretoconjunctivitis 角结膜炎

视网膜 retina

retin(o)   retinitis 视网膜炎；retinoma 视网膜细胞瘤

视觉 vision

opia   diplopia 复视；amblyopia 弱视；myopia 近视

皮肤 skin

dermat(o)   dermatitis 皮炎；dermatofibroma 皮肤纤维瘤

耳 ear

auricul(o)   auricula 耳廓；auricular 耳的

听觉，听力 hearing

audi(o)   audiology 听力学；audiogenic 听原性的

acou   acoustic 听的；acouasm 幻听；

嗅觉 smell

osm(o)   hyperosmia 嗅觉过敏；hyposmia 嗅觉迟钝

olfact(o)   olfactory 嗅觉的；olfactology 嗅觉学

味觉 taste

geusi(o)   hypogeusia 味觉减退；allotriogeusia 味觉异常

gust(o)

肌肉与骨骼系统

肌肉 muscle

muscul(o)   musculocutaneous 肌皮的；musculotendinous 肌腱

my   myocardium 心肌层；myoglobin 肌红蛋白

骨 bone

osse(o)   ossifying 骨化的

oste(o)   osteoarthritis 骨关节炎

软骨 cartilage

chondr(o) perichondrium 软骨膜；chondroma 软骨瘤

韧带 ligament

ligament(o) ligamentous 韧带的；ligamentopexis 圆韧带固定术

腱 tendon

ten(o) tendon 肌腱

tend(o) myotendinous 肌腱的

骨骼 skeleton

skelet(o) skeletal 骨骼的；skeletin 骨骼蛋白

肋骨 rib

cost(o) intercostals 肋间的；subcostal 肋下的

坐骨 ischium

ischi(o) ischium 坐骨；ischiofemoral 坐骨股骨的

椎骨 vertebra

vertebr(o) prevertebral 椎前的；vertebroarterial 椎动脉的

髌骨 patella

patella(o) patellar 髌骨的；patellopexy 髌骨固定术

滑液，滑膜 synovia

synovia(o) synovitis 滑液炎；synovectomy 滑膜切除术；synoviocyte 滑膜细胞

关节 joint

arthr(o) arthritis 关节炎；arthrodesis 关节固定术

细胞与遗传系统

细胞 cell

cyt(o) philcytochrome 细胞色素

cyte hepatocyte 肝细胞

原生质 plasm

plasmcytoplasm 胞浆；plasmamembrane 质膜

核 nut, nucleus

nucle(o) mononuclear 单核的；nucleotide 核苷酸

核糖 ribose

rib(o) ribozyme 核糖酸；ribosome 核蛋白体

色 colour

chrom(o) chromosome 染色体；chromoplast 有色体

基因 gene

gene oncogene 癌基因

gen(o) genetic 基因的

异 different

heter(o) heterophyid 异形的；heterophyidae 异形科

同 same

hom(o) homotomus 同体的；homolog 同源

iso　isotope 同位素

内 within

end(o)　endometrium 子宫内膜；endoparasite 体内寄生虫

单 one

mon(o)　monomeric 单体的；monosome 染色体单体

多 many, much

multi　multiples 多胎；multienzyme 多酶

poly　polypeptide 多肽；multifunctional 多功能的

前 before

pro　prostatic 前列腺的

原 original

prot(o)　protooncogene 原癌基因；protonephron 原肾

组织 tissue

hist(o)　histology 组织学；histidine 组氨酸

皮 derm

thelium　epithelium 腺上皮

thel　epithelization 上皮化

纤维 fiber, fibre

fibr(o)　fibrocyte 纤维细胞；fibrosa 纤维膜

脂肪 fat

lip(o)　lipoma 脂肪瘤；lipopolysaccharide 脂多糖

皮质 cortex

cortic(o)　subcortical 皮下层的；corticosteroid 皮质类固醇

横纹肌 striated muscle

rhabdomy(o)　rhabdomyoma 横纹肌瘤；rhabdomyolvsis 横纹肌溶解
　　　　　　　rhabdomyosarcoma 横纹肌肉瘤

平滑肌 smooth muscle

leiomy(o)　leiomyoma 平滑肌瘤；leiodystonia 平滑肌张力障碍
　　　　　　leiomyofibroma 平滑肌纤维瘤

髓质 medulla

medull(o)　medullitis 骨髓炎；medullectomy 髓质切除术；medulloepithelioma 髓上皮瘤

结 node, knot

nod(o)　nodule 小结；lymphnode 淋巴结

囊 capsule

capusl(o)　capsulitis 囊炎；subcapsular 后囊膜下

叶 lobe, leaf

lob(o)　lobule 小叶；lobectomy 叶切除术

绒毛 villus

vill(o)　villous 绒毛状的；villoma 绒毛瘤

器官 organ

organ(o) organotherapy 器官疗法；organoscopy 内脏镜检查

液体、分泌物与免疫系统

血液 blood

hema hemangioma 血管瘤

hemat(o) hematuria

hem(o) hemolytic 溶血性的；hemodialysis 血透

haem(o) haemoglobin 血红蛋白；haemodialysis 血液透析

haemat(o) haematology 血液学

血浆 plasm

plasm(o) plasma 血浆；plasmin 血浆反应素

血清 serum

ser(o) serological 血清学

orrho orrhotherapy 血清疗法

淋巴 lymph

lymph(o) lymphokine 淋巴因子；lymphocyte 淋巴细胞

乳 milk

lact(o) lactate 乳酸；lactotroph 催乳激素细胞

胆汁 bile

bili biliverdin 胆绿素；d-urobilin d 尿胆素

唾液 spit

saliv(o) salivin 涎液素；salivatory 催涎的

黏液 mucus

blenn(o) blennorrhagia 淋病

myx(o) myxoma 黏液瘤

汗液 sweat

sud(o) sudation 发汗；sudorific 发汗剂

hidr(o) hidradenitis 汗腺炎

粪 feces

fecal(o) fecal 粪便的；fecaloma 粪结；fecal borne 粪传播的

水 water

hydr(o) hydrocephalus 脑积水；hydronephrosis 肾积水

免疫 immunity

immun(o) immunogen 免疫原；immunotherapy 免疫疗法

过敏 allergy

anaphylact(o) anaphylactogen 过敏原；anaphylatoxin 过敏毒素

抗原 antigen

antigen(o) antigenic 抗原的；antigenotherapy 抗原疗法

生物化学系统
蛋白质 protein

protein(o)　proteinuria 蛋白尿症

prote(o)　glycoprotein 糖蛋白

氨基的 amino

amin(o)　aminopeptidase 氨基肽酶；aminotransferase 氨基转移酶

核 nuclear

nucle(o)　nucleotide 核苷酸；nucleoprotein 核蛋白；deoxynucleotide 脱氧核苷酸

脱氧 deoxy

deoxy(o)　deoxyribose 脱氧核糖；deoxynucleotide 脱氧核苷酸

酶 enzyme

enzym(o)　multienzyme 多酶的

zym(o)　zymogenic 发酵菌的，酶原的

糖 sugar

sacchar　polysaccharide 聚糖；oligosaccharide 低聚糖

葡萄糖 glucose

gluc(o)　glucokinase 葡萄糖激酶；glucagon 胰高血糖素

glyco

淀粉 starch

amyl(o)　amylase 淀粉酶；amyloid 淀粉状蛋白

胶，胶质 glue

glio　glioma 胶质瘤；gliotoxin 胶霉毒素

胆固醇 cholesterol

cholester(o)　cholesterosis 胆固醇沉着

cholest　cholesteatoma 胆脂瘤

组氨酸 histidine

histidin(o)　histidase 组氨酸酶；histidinuria 组氨酸尿；histidinemia 组氨酸血症

药物系统
药 drug, medicine

pharmac(o)　pharmacology 药理学；biopharmaceutics 生物药剂学
　　　　　　　pharmacokinetics 药物代谢动力学

疗法 treatment

therapy　chemicotherapy 化学疗法；radiotherapy 放射疗法

溶液 solution

solut　solution 溶液；solute 溶质；dissolution 溶解

麻醉 anesthesia

narco　narcotic 麻醉剂；narcosynthesis 麻醉综合法

胰岛 pancreas islets

insul(o)　insulin 胰岛素；insulinoma 胰岛素瘤；insulogenic 胰岛源的

霉菌素 **moldin**

mycin　micinerythromycin 红霉素；gentamicin 庆大霉素

灌肠法 **enema**

clyster　clysisenteroclysis 灌肠剂；coloclysis 结肠灌洗

剂 **agent**

ant　icdepressant 抑制剂；coagulant 凝血剂；antibiotic 抗生素

in　penicillin 青霉素；aspirin 阿司匹林；analgesic 止痛药

抗、反对 **against**

counter(o)　counterirritant 抗刺激剂

contra　contrastimulant 抗兴奋剂

anti　antibody 抗体

ant　antacide 抗酸的；antalgic 镇痛剂

医学生物学、微生物与寄生虫病学系统

微生物 **microorganism**

microbi(o)　microbial 微生物的；microbiologist 微生物学家；microbicidal 杀微生物的

毒 **poison**

toxi(o)　intoxication 中毒

tox(o)　immunotoxin 免疫毒素

细菌 **germ**

bacter(i)　bacteriology 细菌学；bifidobacterium 双歧杆菌

球菌 **coccus**

cocc(o)　coccuscoccobacillus 球杆菌；diplococcus 双球菌

大肠杆菌 **escherichia**

coli　colicin 大肠杆菌素；coliform 大肠杆菌类；colisepticemia 大肠杆菌败血症

沙门菌 **samonellae**

salmonell(o)　salmonelloses（复）沙门菌；salmonella 沙门菌属
　　　　　　　salmonellosis　沙门菌感染

病毒 **virus**

virus　adenovirus 腺病毒；coronavirus 冠状病毒

支原体 **mycoplasma**

mycoplasm(o)　mycoplasma 支原体；mycoplasmal 支原体的

衣原体 **chlamydia**

chlamyd(o)　chlamydia 衣原体；chlamydial 衣原体的；chlamydemia 衣原体血症

真菌 **fungus**

fungi　fungial 真菌的；fungistasis 抑制真菌

曲霉 **aspergillus**

aspergill　aspergillar 曲霉的；aspergilloma 曲霉肿

孢子 **spore**

sporo　sporozoa 孢子虫；sporogony 孢子增殖

寄生 **parasite**

parasit　parasitosis 寄生虫病；parasitism 寄生

蛔虫 **roundworm**

ascari　ascariasis 蛔虫病；ascaricide 杀蛔虫药

毛滴虫 **trichomonad**

trichomona　trichomonal 毛滴虫的；trichomonasis 毛滴虫病

　　　　　　　trichomonacidal 杀毛滴虫剂的

线虫 **eelworm**

nemat(o)　nematode 线虫；nematodiasis 线虫病

蠕虫 **worm**

verm　vermis 蠕虫，蠕虫结构；verminous 蠕虫的

螨 **mite**

acar(o)　acaridiasis 螨病；acaricide 杀螨药

Appendix 5
Commonly Used Medications

Abacavir 阿巴卡韦

Abciximab 阿昔单抗

Acarbose 阿卡波糖

Acebutolol 醋丁洛尔

Acetaminophen 醋氨酚，对乙酰氨基酚

Acetazolamide 乙酰唑胺

Acetic Acid 乙酸，醋酸

Acetohexamide 乙酰苯磺酰环己脲

Acetylcysteine 乙酰半胱氨酸

Acyclovir 阿昔洛韦，无环鸟苷

Adalimumab 阿达木单抗

Adefovir 阿德福韦

Adenosine 腺苷

Albendazole 阿苯达唑，丙硫咪唑

Albumin 清蛋白，白蛋白

Albuterol 舒喘灵，沙丁胺醇

Alclometasone 阿氯米松

Aldesleukin 阿地白介素

Alemtuzumab 阿仑单抗

Alfentanil 阿芬太尼

Alfuzosin 阿夫唑嗪，阿夫佐辛

Alitretinoin 阿利维 A 酸

Allopurinol 别嘌呤醇

Almotriptan 阿莫曲坦

Alosetron 阿洛司琼

Alprazolam 阿普唑仑

Alprostadil 前列地尔

Alteplase 阿替普酶

Altretamine 六甲蜜胺

Aluminum Hydroxide 氢氧化铝

Amantadine　金刚（烷）胺，三环癸胺

Amifostine　阿米斯丁，氨磷丁

Amikacin　丁胺卡那霉素

Amiloride　阿米洛利，氨氯吡脒

Aminocaproic Acid　氨基己酸

Amiodarone　胺碘达隆，胺碘酮

Amitriptyline　阿米替林，阿密曲替林

AmLodipine　氨氯地平，阿洛地平，络活喜

Ammonium Lactate　乳酸铵

Amobarbital　异戊巴比妥

Amphetamine　安非他明

Amoxicillin　阿莫西林，羟氨苄青霉素

Ampicillin　氨比西林，氨苄青霉素

Amphotericin B　两性霉素 B，二性霉素 B

Amyl Nitrite　亚硝酸戊酯

Anagrelide　阿那格雷，氯咪喹酮

Anastrozole　阿那曲唑

Androstenedione　雄（甾）烯二酮

Anidulafungin　阿尼芬净

Anistreplase　复合纤溶酶链激酶

Antipyrine　安替比林

Apomorphine　阿朴吗啡，脱水吗啡

Aprepitant　阿瑞吡坦

Aprotinin　抗蛋白酶肽，抑酶肽

Aripiprazole　阿立哌唑

Articaine　阿替卡因

Ascorbic Acid　抗坏血酸维生素 C

Aspirin　阿司匹林

Astemizole　阿司咪唑，息斯敏

Atazanavir　阿扎那韦

Atenolol　阿替洛尔，氨酰心安

Atorvastatin　阿托伐他汀

Atropine　阿托品，颠茄碱

Azathioprine　（硝基）咪唑硫嘌呤

Azithromycin　阿奇霉素

Aztreonam　噻肟单酰胺菌素，氨曲南

Barium Sulfate　硫酸钡

Bacitracin　杆菌肽，枯草杆菌抗生素

Basiliximab　巴利昔单抗

Baclofen　巴氯芬，氯苯氨丁酸

Beclomethasone　氯地米松，倍氯米松

Benazepril　贝那普利

Benztropine　苯托品

Benzphetamine　苄非他明，甲苯丙胺

Betamethasone　倍他米松

Betaxolol　倍他索洛尔

Bevacizumab　贝伐单抗

Bethanechol　乌拉胆碱，氨甲酰甲胆碱

Bexarotene　贝沙罗汀

Bimatoprost　比马前列素

Bisoprolol　比索洛尔

Bismuth Subsalicylate　次水杨酸铋，水杨酸亚铋

Bivalirudin　比伐卢定

Bleomycin　博来霉素，争光霉素

Boric Acid　硼酸

Botulinum Toxin　肉毒杆菌毒素

Bretylium　溴苄胺

Bromocriptine　溴麦角环肽，溴麦角隐亭

Brompheniramine　溴苯那敏

Budesonide　布地奈德

Bumetanide　丁尿胺，布美他尼

Bupivacaine　丁哌卡因

Buprenorphine　丁丙诺啡

Bupropion　安非拉酮，丁基丙酸苯

Buspirone　丁螺环酮

Busulfan　白消安，甲磺酸丁二醇二酯

Butoconazole　布康唑

Butabarbital　仲丁巴比妥，另丁巴比妥

Butorphanol　布托啡诺

Calcitonin　降血钙素

Calcium Salts　钙盐

Calcium　钙

Calcium Carbonate　碳酸钙

Candesartan　坎地沙坦

Capsaicin　辣椒素，辣椒苦

Captopril　甲巯丙脯酸

Capecitabine　卡培他滨

Carbamazepine　卡巴咪嗪，痛痉宁，痛可宁，立痛定

Carbenicillin　羧苄青霉素

Carbetapentane　咳必清，喷托维林

Carbidopa　卡比多巴，甲基多巴肼

Carbinoxamine　卡比沙明

Carboplatin　卡铂，碳铂，卡波铂

Carteolol　喹酮心安，卡替洛尔

Carvedilol　卡维地洛，卡维洛尔，卡文心安，卡地洛尔

Caspofungin　卡泊芬净

Castor Oil　蓖麻油

Cefaclor　氯氨苄青霉素，头孢克洛

Cefadroxil　头孢羟氨苄，羟氨苄头孢菌素，头孢拉定

Cefazolin　唑啉头孢菌素，先锋霉素 V

Cefdinir　头孢地尼

Cefditoren　头孢妥仑酯，头孢托仑

Cefepime　头孢平，头孢吡肟

Cefixime　头孢克肟，世福素

Cefotaxime　头孢噻肟，氨噻肟头孢菌素

Cefoperazone　头孢哌酮，头孢氧哌唑，头孢氧哌羟苯唑，先锋必

Cefotetan　头孢替坦

Cefoxitin　头孢西丁，头孢甲氧霉素

Cefpodoxime　头孢泊肟，头孢泊肟酯

Cefpodoxime　头孢泊肟

Cefprozil　头孢罗齐，赛夫罗秀，头孢丙烯

Ceftazidime　头孢他定，头孢塔齐定，凯复定，凯福定

Ceftibuten　头孢布坦，头孢丁烯

Ceftizoxime　头孢唑肟

Ceftriaxone　头孢曲松钠

Cefuroxime　头孢呋辛，头孢呋肟

Celecoxib　塞来考昔，塞来昔布

Cephalexin　头孢氨苄，苯甘头孢菌素，头孢菌素 IV

Cephalothin　头孢菌素，先锋霉素

Cephradine　头孢拉啶，环己烯胺头孢菌素

Cerivastatin　西立伐他汀

Cetirizine　西替立嗪

Cetrorelix　西曲瑞克

Cetuximab　西妥昔单抗

Cevimeline　西维美林

Charcoal　木炭，活性炭

Chloral Hydrate　水合氯醛

Chlorambucil　苯丁酸氮芥，瘤可宁

Chloramphenicol　氯霉素

Chlordiazepoxide　甲氨二氮，利眠宁

Chloroprocaine 氯普鲁卡因

Chlorhexidine 洗必泰，双氯苯双胍己烷

Chloroquine 氯喹

Chlorothiazide 氯噻，氯噻嗪

Chlorpromazine 氯丙嗪

Chlorpheniramine 氯苯吡胺，扑尔敏

Chlorpropamide 氯磺丙脲

Chlorthalidone 氯噻酮

Cholestyramine 消胆胺

Choline Salicylate 胆碱水杨酸盐

Chondroitin 软骨素

Cidofovir 西多福韦

Cimetidine 甲氰咪胍，甲腈咪胍

Cilostazol 西洛他唑

Cinoxacin 西诺沙星

Ciprofloxacin 环丙沙星，丙氟哌，悉复欢

Cisapride 西沙比利

Cisplatin 顺铂，顺氯氨铂，氯氨铂

Citric Acid 柠檬酸

Clarithromycin 克拉仙霉素，甲基红霉素，克拉仙，克拉红霉素

Clemastine 氯马斯汀，克立马汀

Clindamycin 氯林可霉素，克林霉素

Clobetasol 氯倍他索

Clofazimine 氯苯吩嗪

Clofibrate 降固醇酸，安妥明

Clomipramine 氯米帕明，氯丙咪嗪

Clonazepam 氯硝西泮，氯硝安定

Clonidine 氯压定，可乐宁，可乐亭

Clopidogrel 氯吡格雷，克拉匹多

Clotrimazole 克霉唑，氯三苯甲咪唑

Clozapine 氯氮平

Cocaine 可卡因

Codeine 可待因

Colchicine 秋水仙碱，秋水仙素

Cortisone 可的松，肾上腺皮质酮

Corticotropin 促肾上腺皮质激素，亲皮质素

Cromolyn Sodium 色甘酸钠

Cyanocobalamin 维生素 B_{12}，氰钴维生素

Cyclophosphamide 环磷酰胺

Cycloserine 环丝氨酸

Cyclosporine　环孢霉素

Cyproheptadine　赛庚啶，二苯环庚啶

Econazole　益康唑

Edrophonium　氯化腾喜龙

Eletriptan　依立曲坦

Enalapril　恩纳普利，乙丙脯氨酸，依那普利

Enoxaparin　依诺肝素

Entacapone　恩他卡朋

Entecavir　恩替卡韦

Ephedra　麻黄属植物

Ephedrine　麻黄碱，麻黄素

Epinephrine　肾上腺素

Epoprostenol　依前列醇，依前列素

Epoetin Alfa　阿法依泊汀，促红细胞生成素

Ergocalciferol　钙化醇，维生素 D_2

Ergoloid Mesylates　二氢麦角毒甲磺酸盐

Ergonovine　麦角新碱

Ergotamine　麦角胺

Erythromycin　红霉素

Ertapenem　厄他培南，碳青霉烯类

Esmolol　艾司洛尔

Esomeprazole　索美拉唑，埃索美拉唑

Estazolam　艾司唑仑，舒乐安定

Estradiol　雌二醇，强力求偶素

Ethambutol　乙胺丁醇

Ethionamide　乙硫异烟胺

Ethosuximide　乙琥胺

Ethotoin　乙基苯妥英，乙妥英

Etidocaine　依替卡因

Exemestane　依西美坦

Ezetimibe　依泽替米贝

Famciclovir　泛昔洛韦

Famotidine　法莫替丁

Felodipine　非洛地平

Fentanyl　芬太尼

Fexofenadine　非索非那定

Fluconazole　氟康唑，大扶康

Flucytosine　氟胞嘧啶

Fludrocortisone　氟氢可的松

Flumazenil　氟马西尼，氟甲泽宁

Flunisolide　氟尼缩松

Fluocinolone　氟轻松，丙酮化氟新龙

Fluorometholone　氟米龙

Fluorouracil　氟尿嘧啶，氟二氧嘧啶

Flurandrenolide　氟氢缩松

Fluoxetine　氟西汀，百忧解，盐酸氟西汀

Fluticasone　氟地松，氟替卡松

Folic Acid　叶酸，维生素 B

Follitropin　促滤泡素，促卵泡素

Fosinopril　福森普利，福辛普利

Furazolidone　呋喃唑酮，痢特灵

Furosemide　呋喃苯胺酸，速尿

Gabapentin　加巴喷丁

Ganciclovir　羟甲基无环鸟苷，更昔洛韦

Garlic　大蒜，蒜头

Gatifloxacin　加替沙星

Gemifloxacin　吉米沙星

Gentamicin　庆大霉素

Glimepiride　格列美脲

Glipizide　格列吡嗪

Glucagon　胰高血糖素

Glyburide　优降糖，格列本脲

Glycopyrrolate　格隆铵，胃长宁

Gramicidin　短杆菌肽

Granisetron　格拉司琼，康泉

Griseofulvin　灰黄霉素

Haloperidol　氟哌啶醇，氟哌丁苯

Heparin　肝磷脂，肝素

Hydralazine　肼苯哒嗪，肼太嗪

Hydrochlorothiazide　二氢氯噻，双氢克尿塞

Hydrocodone　氢可酮，二氢可待因酮

Hydrocortisone　氢化可的松，皮质醇

Hydromorphone　氢吗啡酮

Hydroxychloroquine　羟化氯喹

Hydroxyzine　羟嗪

Hyoscyamine　莨菪碱，天仙子胺

Ibuprofen　布洛芬，异丁苯丙酸

Ibutilide　伊布利特

Ifosfamide　异环磷酰胺

Idarubicin　去甲氧基柔红霉素

Iloprost　伊洛前列素

Imatinib　伊马替尼，格列卫，加以域

Imipenem　亚胺培南

Imipramine　丙咪嗪

Inamrinone　氨力农

Indapamide　吲达胺，长效降压片，吲满酰胺，吲达帕胺，寿比山

Indinavir　印地那韦

Indomethacin　消炎痛

Infliximab　英夫利昔单抗

Insulin Aspart　门冬胰岛素

Insulin Detemir　地特胰岛素

Insulin Glargine　甘精胰岛素

Insulin Lispro　赖脯胰岛素

Interferon　干扰素

Ipecac　吐根，吐根树

Ipratropium　异丙托铵

Iron Dextran　右旋糖酐铁

Isocarboxazid　异唑酰肼，闷可乐

Isoproterenol　异丙（去甲）肾上腺素

Isophane Insulin　中效胰岛素，低精锌胰岛素

Isradipine　依拉地平

Isosorbide Dinitrate　异山梨醇硝酸酯，消心痛

Itraconazole　伊曲康唑

Ivermectin　伊佛霉素

Ketamine　克他命，氯胺酮

Ketoconazole　酮康唑

Ketoprofen　酮基布洛芬，优布芬

Ketorolac　酮咯酸

Lactase　乳糖分解酵素

Lactobacillus　乳酸菌；乳杆菌属

Lactulose　半乳糖苷果糖

Lamivudine　拉米夫定，拉美夫定

Lamotrigine　拉莫三嗪，乐命达

Lansoprazole　南索拉唑，兰索拉唑

Lercanidipine　乐卡地平

Lente Insulin　慢胰岛素锌悬液

Letrozole　来曲唑，来罗唑

Levalbuterol　左旋沙丁胺醇

Levetiracetam　左乙拉西坦

Levobetaxolol　左倍他洛尔

Levodopa　左旋多巴

Levofloxacin　左氧氟沙星

Levothyroxine　左旋甲状腺素

Lidocaine　利多卡因

Lincomycin　林肯霉素，洁霉素

Linezolid　利奈唑胺，利奈唑酮

Liotrix　复方甲状腺素

Lisinopril　赖诺普利，苯丁酸赖脯酸

Lithium　锂

Lomefloxacin　洛美沙星，美沙星

Lomustine　环己亚硝脲，罗氮芥

Lopinavir　洛匹那韦

Loracarbef　氯拉卡比，洛拉卡比

Loratadine　氯雷他定

Losartan　氯沙坦

Lorazepam　劳拉西泮，氯羟去甲安定

Loxapine　洛沙平

Lovastatin　洛伐他汀，洛弗斯塔特因

Magaldrate　氢氧化镁铝

Magnesium Citrate　柠檬酸镁

Magnesium Hydroxide　氢氧化镁

Magnesium Salicylate　水杨酸镁

Mannitol　甘露醇

Maprotiline　马普替林

Mebendazole　甲苯咪唑，甲苯哒唑

Mechlorethamine　二氯甲基二乙胺，氮芥

Meclizine　美其敏，敏克静

Melatonin　褪黑激素

Mefloquine　甲氟喹

Megestrol　甲地孕酮

Melphalan　美法仑，左旋溶肉瘤素

Meperidine　哌替啶，杜冷丁

Mephobarbital　甲基苯巴比妥

Meprobamate　安宁，眠尔通

Meropenem　倍能（美罗培南粉针剂）

Mesoridazine　美索哒嗪

Mestranol　炔雌醇甲醚

Metaproterenol　间羟异丙肾上腺

Metaxalone　美他沙酮

Metformin　甲福明，二甲双胍

Methadone   美沙酮

Methazolamide   美舍唑咪，甲醋唑胺

Methimazole   甲巯基咪唑，他巴唑

Methocarbamol   美索巴莫

Methotrexate   甲氨蝶呤，氨甲蝶呤

Methoxsalen   甲氧沙林，花椒毒素

Methscopolamine   甲基东莨菪碱

Methoxyflurane   甲氧氟烷，二氟二氯乙基甲醚

Methyldopa   甲基多巴

Methyclothiazide   甲氯噻嗪，因德降，利尿散

Methylphenidate   利他灵

Methylprednisolone   甲强龙，甲基强的松龙

Metipranolol   美替洛尔，三甲苯心安

Methyltestosterone   甲基睾（丸）酮，甲睾丸素

Metoclopramide   灭吐灵，胃复安

Metolazone   美托拉宗，甲苯喹唑磺胺

Metoprolol   美托洛尔

Metronidazole   灭滴灵，甲硝哒唑

Mezlocillin   美洛西林

Mibefradil   咪拉地尔

Micafungin   米卡芬净

Miconazole   霉康唑，咪康唑

Midazolam   咪达唑仑

Midodrine   米多君，甲氧安福林

Mifepristone   米非司酮

Miglitol   米格列醇

Miglustat   美格鲁特

Milrinone   米利酮，二联吡啶酮，米力农

Mirtazapine   米尔塔扎平

Misoprostol   迷索前列醇

Mitomycin   丝裂霉素

Mitotane   米托坦

Moexipril   莫昔普利

Mometasone   莫米松

Morphine   吗啡

Montelukast   孟鲁司特

Moxifloxacin   莫西沙星

Mupirocin   莫匹罗星

Nafcillin   新青霉素Ⅲ，萘夫西林

Nadolol   纳多洛尔，康格尔，康格多

Nalbuphine　纳布啡

Nalmefene　纳美芬

Naloxone　纳洛酮，烯丙羟吗啡酮

Naltrexone　环丙甲羟二羟吗啡酮

Naproxen　甲氧萘丙酸，萘普生

Naratriptan　那拉曲坦

Nateglinide　那格列奈，那格列胺

Nedocromil　萘多罗米

Nelfinavir　那非那韦

Neomycin　新霉素

Neostigmine　新斯的明

Nepafenac　奈帕芬胺

Nesiritide　奈西立肽

Nevirapine　奈韦拉平

Niacin　烟酸的商品名，尼亚新

Nicardipine　硝吡胺甲酯

Nicotine　尼古丁，烟碱

Nifedipine　硝苯吡啶，利心平，心痛定

Nilutamide　安得乐

Nimodipine　尼莫地平，硝苯吡酯

Nitric Oxide　氧化一氮

Nisoldipine　尼索地平，硝苯异丙啶

Nitrofurantoin　呋喃妥英，呋喃咀啶

Nitroglycerin　硝化甘油

Norepinephrine　去甲肾上腺素

Nitroprusside　硝普盐，硝基氢氰酸盐

Norethindrone　炔诺酮

Norfloxacin　诺氟沙星，氟哌酸

Norfloxacin　诺氟沙星，氟哌酸

Nortriptyline　去甲替林，去甲阿米替林

Nystatin　制霉菌素，制真菌素

Ofloxacin　氧氟沙星，可乐必妥，康泰必妥，泰利必妥

Olanzapine　奥氮平，奥兰氮平

Olmesartan　奥美沙坦

Olopatadine　奥洛他定

Omeprazole　奥美拉唑，沃必唑，洛赛克

Omalizumab　奥马佐单抗

Ondansetron　奥坦西隆，枢复宁

Oprelvekin　奥普瑞白介素

Orphenadrine　邻甲苯海拉明

Oseltamivir   奥塞米韦

Oxacillin   苯甲异唑青霉素，新青霉素 II

Oxaprozin   丙嗪，苯丙酸

Oxazepam   去甲羟基安定，氯羟氧二氮

Oxcarbazepine   奥卡西平

Oxiconazole   奥昔康唑，醋苯苄肟唑

Oxybutynin   奥昔布宁

Oxycodone   氧可酮

Oxymorphone   氧吗啡酮

Oxytocin   后叶催产素

Paclitaxel   紫杉醇

Palonosetron   帕洛诺司琼

Pancreatin   胰液素

Pancrelipase   胰脂肪酶

Pantoprazole   泮托拉唑

Pantothenic Acid   泛酸（维生素 B_3）

Papaverine   罂粟碱

Para Aminobenzoic Acid   对氨基苯（甲）酸

Paricalcitol   帕立骨化醇

Paromomycin   巴龙霉素

Paroxetine   氟苯哌苯醚，帕罗西丁

Pegaspargase   天门冬酰胺酶，培加帕酶

Pegfilgrastim   乙二醇化非格司亭

Pemetrexed   培美曲塞

Pemirolast   哌罗来斯

Penbutolol   喷布洛尔

Penciclovir   喷西洛维

Penicillamine   青霉胺

Penicillin   青霉素

Pentamidine   潘他米丁

Pentobarbital   戊巴比妥

Pentazocine   戊唑辛，镇痛新

Pentostatin   喷司他丁

Pergolide   培高利特，硫丙麦角林

Perindopril   哌道普利，哌林多普利

Perphenazine   奋乃静，羟哌氯丙嗪

Phenelzine   苯乙肼

Phenobarbital   镇静安眠剂

Phentermine   苯丁胺

Phenylephrine   苯肾上腺素

Phenytoin　苯妥英，二苯乙内酰脲

Phenylpropanolamine　苯丙醇胺

Phosphorus Salts　磷盐

Physostigmine　毒扁豆碱

Pilocarpine　匹鲁卡品，毛果芸香碱

Pimecrolimus　吡美莫司

Pimozide　哌迷清，双氟苯丁哌啶

Pindolol　心得乐，心得静

Pioglitazone　吡格列酮

Piperacillin　哌拉西林，氧哌嗪青霉素

Pleconaril　普来可那立

Plicamycin　光神霉素，光辉霉素

Polymyxin B　多黏霉素 B，多黏菌素

Posaconazole　泊沙康唑

Potassium Iodide　碘化钾

Potassium Salts　钾盐

Pramipexole　普拉克索

Pralidoxime　磷定；1- 甲 -2- 吡啶甲醛肟盐

PramLintide　普兰林肽

Pravastatin　帕伐他汀，哌伐它停，泼瓦停

Praziquantel　吡喹酮

Prazosin　哌唑嗪

Prednisone　泼尼松，强的松

Prednisolone　脱氢皮质（甾）醇，氢化波尼松

Prilocaine　丙胺卡因

Primidone　普里米酮，扑痫酮

Probenecid　丙磺舒，羧苯磺丙胺

Procarbazine　甲基苄肼，甲苄肼

Procainamide　普鲁卡因酰胺

Procaine　普鲁卡因

Progesterone　孕酮，黄体酮

Promethazine　普鲁米近，异丙嗪

Propafenone　丙胺苯丙酮

Propantheline　丙胺太林，普鲁本辛

Propofol　异丙酚，丙泊酚

Propoxyphene　丙氧芬

Propranolol　心得安

Propylthiouracil　丙基硫尿嘧啶

Protamine　（鱼）精蛋白

Protriptyline　普罗替林

Pseudoephedrine　假麻黄碱

Psyllium　（洋）车前草

Pyrantel　噻嘧啶，噻吩嘧啶

Pyrazinamide　吡嗪酰胺

Pyridostigmine　吡啶斯的明

Pyridoxine　维生素 B_6

Pyrimethamine　乙嘧啶，息疟定

Quinapril　喹那普利

Quinidine　奎尼丁

Ramipril　雷米普利

Ranibizumab　单抗

Ranitidine　雷尼替丁

Reboxetine　瑞波西汀

Regular Insulin　普通胰岛素，胰岛素

Remifentanil　雷米芬太尼

Repaglinide　瑞格列奈

Reserpine　利血平

Reteplase　瑞替普酶

Ribavirin　三（氮）唑核苷，病毒唑

Riboflavin　核黄素

Rifabutin　利福布丁

Rifampin　利福平

Rifaximin　利福昔明

Rifapentine　利福喷丁，环戊去甲利福平

Rimantadine　金刚烷乙胺

Risperidone　利哌利酮，利哌酮

Ritonavir　利托那韦

Rituximab　利妥昔单抗

Rizatriptan　利扎曲坦

Rivastigmine　利凡斯的明，利伐斯的明

Rofecoxib　罗非考昔

Ropivacaine　罗哌卡因

Rosuvastatin　罗苏伐他汀

Rosiglitazone　罗西格列酮，罗格列酮

Salmeterol　沙美特罗

Saquinavir　沙奎那韦

Scopolamine　东莨菪碱

Secobarbital　司可巴比妥，速可眠

Senna　番泻叶

Sertaconazole　丝他康唑

Sertraline　舍曲林

Sildenafil　昔多芬，伟哥，西地那非

Simethicone　二甲基硅油

Simvastatin　辛伐他汀

Sodium Bicarbonate　碳酸氢钠，小苏打

Sodium Fluoride　氟化钠

Sodium Iodide　碘化钠

Sodium Lactate　乳酸钠

Sodium bicarbonate　碳酸氢钠，小苏打

Somatropin　促生长激素

Sorafenib　索拉非尼，多吉美

Sotalol　甲磺胺心定，心得怡

Sparfloxacin　施怕沙星

Spectinomycin　奇放线菌素，奇霉素

Spirapril　螺普利

Spironolactone　安体舒通，螺内酯

Stavudine　司他夫定

Streptokinase　链激酶，溶栓酶

Streptomycin　链霉素

Sucralfate　硫糖铝，胃溃宁

Sufentanil　芬太尼，舒芬太尼

Sulconazole　硫康唑，氯苄硫咪唑

Sulfacetamide　磺胺醋酰，乙酰磺胺

Sulfadiazine　磺胺嘧啶

Sulfisoxazole　磺胺二甲基异噁唑，甘特里辛

Sulfamethoxazole　磺胺甲唑，磺胺甲基异噁唑，新明磺，新诺明

Sumatriptan　舒马曲坦

Tadalafil　他达拉非

Tamsulosin　坦（索）洛新

Telithromycin　泰利霉素

Temazepam　羟基安定

Temozolomide　替莫唑胺

Tenecteplase　替奈普酶

Terazosin　特拉唑嗪

Tenofovir　替诺福韦

Terbutaline　间羟叔丁肾上腺素

Tetracycline　四环素

Theophylline　茶碱

Thiamine　硫胺（维生素 B_1）

Thioguanine　硫鸟嘌呤

Thiopental 戊硫代巴比妥

Thioridazine 甲硫哒嗪，硫醚嗪

Thrombin 凝血酶

Thyrotropin Alfa 促甲状腺素 α

Tigecycline 替加环素

Ticarcillin α 替卡西林，羟基噻吩青霉素

Timolol 噻吗洛尔

Tinidazole 磺甲硝咪唑

Tipranavir 替拉那韦

Tobramycin 托普霉素

Tolazamide 甲磺氮草脲，甲磺吖庚脲

Tolbutamide 甲苯磺丁脲，甲糖宁

Tolcapone 托卡朋

Tolmetin 甲苯酰吡啶乙酸

Torsemide 托塞米

Trandolapril 群多普利

Trastuzumab 曲妥单抗，群司珠单抗

Trazodone 曲唑酮，氯哌三唑酮

Treprostinil 曲前列环素

Tretinoin 维生素 A 酸，视黄酸

Triamcinolone 去炎松

Triamterene 三氨蝶呤，氨苯蝶啶

Trihexyphenidyl 安坦

Trimethoprim 甲氧苄氨嘧啶

Trimetrexate 曲美沙特

Troglitazone 曲格列酮

Trovafloxacin 曲伐沙星

Tubocurarine 筒箭毒碱

Urokinase 尿激酶

Ultralente Insulin 特慢胰岛素

Valacyclovir 伐昔洛韦

Valdecoxib 伐地考昔

Valganciclovir 缬更昔洛韦

Valproic Acid 丙戊酸，2- 丙基戊酸

Valsartan 缬沙坦

Vancomycin 万古霉素

Venlafaxine 文拉法辛

Vasopressin 后叶加压素，抗利尿激素

Vinblastine 长春碱

Vincristine 长春新碱

Vinorelbine   长春瑞滨

Vitamin   维生素

Voriconazole   伏立康唑

Warfarin   华法林

Zafirlukast   扎鲁司特

Zanamivir   扎那米韦

Ziconotide   齐考诺肽

Zidovudine   齐多呋定，叠氮胸苷

Zinc Oxide   氧化锌

Ziprasidone   齐拉西酮

Zolmitriptan   佐米曲坦

Zolpidem   唑吡坦，佐尔吡啶

Appendix 6
References

1. 2005 American Heart Association Guidelines for Cardiopulmonary Resuscitation and Emergency Cardiovascular Care, 2005.

2. 2015 American Heart Association Guidelines for Cardiopulmonary Resuscitation and Emergency Cardiovascular Care, 2015.

3. Akyildiz Z.I., Ergene O. Frequency of angina and quality of life in outpatients with stable coronary artery disease in Turkey: insights from the PULSE study [J]. Acta Cardiol, 2014.

4. Alonso J.J., Muñiz J., Gómez-Doblas J.J.,et al. Prevalence of stable angina in Spain. Results of the OFRECE study [J]. Rev Esp Cardiol (Engl Ed), 2015.

5. American Heart Association in collaboration with International Liaison Committee on Resuscitation. Guidelines 2000 for Cardiopulmonary Resuscitation and Emergency Cardiovascular Care: International Consensus on Science. Circulation, 2000.

6. American Nurses Association. Nursing: Scope and Standards of Practice [M]. Washington, DC: ANA, 2004.

7. Berman, A., Snyder, S., Kozier, Erb, et al. Fundamentals of Nursing: Concepts, Process, and Practice [M]. 9th ed. Upper Saddle River, NJ: Pearson, 2012.

8. Bochkareva E.V., Kukurina E.V., Voronina V.P., et al. Painless myocardial ischemia at various blood pressure levels in patients with effort angina (J-shaped relationship) [J]. Kardiologiia, 2005.

9. Bruijn R.F.D., Bos M.J., Portegies M.L., et al. The potential for prevention of dementia across two decades: the prospective, population-based Rotterdam Study [J]. Bmc Medicine, 2015.

10. Cardiopulmonary resuscitation [J]. JAMA, 1966.

11. Clemen-Stone, S., Eigsti D.G.& McGuire S.L. Comprehensive Community Health nursing: Family, Aggregate & Community Practice [M]. 4th ed. St. Louis, MO: Mosby Year Book, 1995.

12. Codolosa J.N., Acharjee S., Figueredo V.M., et al. Update on ranolazine in the management of angina [J]. Vasc Health Risk Management, 2014.

13. Craig P., Dolan P., Drew K., et al. Nursing Assessment, Plan of Care, and Patient Education: The Foundation of Patient Care [M]. Lancaster, PA: HCPro, 2006.

14. Dalton J.A. & McNaull F.A. Call for standardizing the clinical rating of pain intensity using a 0 to 10 rating scale [J]. Cancer Nursing, 1986.

15. Danis D.M., Blansfield J.S., Gervasini A.A. Handbook of Clinical Trauma Care: The First Hour [M]. 4th ed. St Louis, Mo: Mosby Elsevier, 2007.

16. Dillon, P. M. Nursing Health Assessment: A Critical Thinking, Case Studies Approach [M]. Philadelphia, PA: F. A. Davis Company, 2007.

17. Donahue M.P. Nursing: the Finest Art: an illustrated istory [M]. St. Louis, MO: CV. Mosby, 1985.

18. Field J.M., Hazinski M.F., Sayre M.R., et al. Part 1: executive summary: 2010 American Heart Association Guidelines for Cardiopulmonary Resuscitation and Emergency Cardiovascular Care [J]. Circulation, 2010.

19. Fihn S.D., Gardin J.M., Abrams J., et al. 2012 ACCF/AHA/ACP/AATS/PCNA/SCAI/ STS. Guideline for the diagnosis and management of patients with stable ischemic heart disease: a report of the American College of Cardiology Foundation/American Heart Association Task Force on Practice Guidelines, and the American College of Physicians, American Association for Thoracic Surgery, Preventive Cardiovascular Nurses Association, Society for Cardiovascular Angiography and Interventions, and Society of Thoracic Surgeons [J]. J Am Coll Cardiol, 2012.

20. Go A.S., Mozaffarian D., Roger V.L., et al. Heart disease and stroke statistics-2013 update: a report from the American Heart Association [J]. Circulation, 2013.

21. Guidelines for cardiopulmonary resuscitation and emergency cardiac care. Emergency Cardiac Care Committee and Subcommittees, American Heart Association [J]. JAMA, 1992.

22. Henderson V. The Nature of Nursing [M]. New York: Macmillan, 1966.

23. https://eccguidelines.heart.org/index.php/circulation/cpr-ecc-guidelines-2/part-1-executive-summary/. Accessed December 25, 2015.

24. Ignatavicius D.D. & Workman M.L. Medical surgical nursing: patient centered collaborative care [M]. 6th ed. Saint Louis, MO: Saunders, 2010.

25. International Association for the Study of Pain. Pain terms: a list with definitions and notes on usage, Recommended by the IASP Subcommittee on Taxonomy. Pain, 1979.

26. International Council of Nurses. The ICN Definition of Nursing. Geneva: ICN [OB/OL]. http://www.icn.ch/about-icn/icn-definition-of-nursing/.

27. Macer. D.R.J. Bioethethics for Informed Citizens Across Cultures [M]. Eubios Ethics Institute, 2004.

28. Manuel Praga & Angel Sevillano. Changes in the etiology, clinical presentation and management of acute interstitial nephritis, an increasingly common cause of acute kidney injury [J]. Nephrol Dial Transplant, 2015.

29. Mary L. Dolan. Living with Alzheimer's disease: an examination of caregiver coping mechanisms[D]. Ohio: The Honors Tutorial College Ohio University, 2010.

30. McCaffery M. & Pasero C. Pain: Clinical Manual [M]. ed2, St Louis: Mosby, 1999.

31. McGillion M., Croxford R., Watt-Watson J., et al. Cost of illness for chronic stable angina patients enrolled in a self-management education trial [J]. Can J Cardiol, 2008.

32. National Research Council. Accidental Death and Disability: The Neglected Disease of Modern Society [M]. Washington DC: The National Academies Press, 1966.

33. Neilson E.G. Tubulointerstitial diseases. In: Goldman L, Ausiello D, eds. Cecil Medicine [M]. 23rd ed. Philadelphia, Pa: Saunders Elsevier, 2007.

34. Nies M.A. & McEwen M. Community Health Nursing: Promoting the Health of Populations [M]. 3rd ed. Philadelphia, PA: W.B. Saunders, 2001.

35. Nightingale F. Notes on nursing: What It Is and What It Is Not [M]. London: Harrison, 1859.

36. Olanrewaju O., Clare L., Barnes L., et al. A multimodal approach to dementia prevention: a report from the Cambridge Institute of Public Health [J]. Alzheimers & Dementia Translational Research & Clinical Interventions, 2015.

37. Peisah, C. & Brodaty, H. Managing Alzheimer's disease the role of the GP [J]. Medicine Today, 2005.

38. Potter P.A., Perry A.G. Fundamentals of Nursing [M]. 7th ed. Saint Louis, 2009.

39. Rutty J.E. The nature of philosophy of science, theory and knowledge relating to nursing and professionalism [J]. Journal of Advanced Nursing, 1998.

40. Shaw G. Participate in dementia prevention: volunteering for clinical trials is a meaningful way to push research forward on Alzheimer's disease and dementia. Here are a few studies to consider [J]. Neurology Now, 2015.

41. Silverman M.E. William Heberden and some account of a disorder of the breast [J]. Clin Cardio, 1987.

42. Smeltzer, S.C., Bare, B.G., Hinkle,J.L., et al. Brunner and Suddarth's Textbook of Medical-surgical Nursing [M]. 11th ed. Philadelphia, PA: Lippincott Williams & Wilkins, 2006.

43. Smith L.S. Is nursing an academic discipline [J]. Nursing Forum, 2000.

44. Sole M.L., Klein D.G., Moseley M.J. Introduction to Critical Care Nursing [M]. 5th ed. St. Louis, Mo: Saunders/Elsevier, 2009.

45. Solomon A., Soininen H. Dementia: risk prediction models in dementia prevention [J]. Nature Reviews Neurology, 2015.

46. Standards and guidelines for cardiopulmonary resuscitation (CPR) and emergency cardiac care (ECC). National Academy of Sciences - National Research Council [J]. JAMA, 1986.

47. Standards and guidelines for cardiopulmonary resuscitation (CPR) and emergency cardiac care (ECC) [J]. JAMA, 1980.

48. Standards for cardiopulmonary resuscitation (CPR) and emergency cardiac care (ECC). 3. Advanced life support [J]. JAMA, 1974.

49. Tang E.Y.H., Harrison S.L., Albanese E., et al. Dietary interventions for prevention of dementia in people with mild cognitive impairment [J]. Cochrane Database of Systematic Reviews, 2015.

50. Tintinalli J.E., Stapczynski J.S. Tintinallis Emergency Medicine [M]. 7th ed. New York: McGraw Hill, 2011.

全国中医药行业高等教育"十四五"规划教材

全国高等中医药院校规划教材（第十一版）

教材目录（第一批）

注：凡标☆号者为"核心示范教材"。

（一）中医学类专业

序号	书　名	主　编		主编所在单位	
1	中国医学史	郭宏伟	徐江雁	黑龙江中医药大学	河南中医药大学
2	医古文	王育林	李亚军	北京中医药大学	陕西中医药大学
3	大学语文	黄作阵		北京中医药大学	
4	中医基础理论☆	郑洪新	杨　柱	辽宁中医药大学	贵州中医药大学
5	中医诊断学☆	李灿东	方朝义	福建中医药大学	河北中医学院
6	中药学☆	钟赣生	杨柏灿	北京中医药大学	上海中医药大学
7	方剂学☆	李　冀	左铮云	黑龙江中医药大学	江西中医药大学
8	内经选读☆	翟双庆	黎敬波	北京中医药大学	广州中医药大学
9	伤寒论选读☆	王庆国	周春祥	北京中医药大学	南京中医药大学
10	金匮要略☆	范永升	姜德友	浙江中医药大学	黑龙江中医药大学
11	温病学☆	谷晓红	马　健	北京中医药大学	南京中医药大学
12	中医内科学☆	吴勉华	石　岩	南京中医药大学	辽宁中医药大学
13	中医外科学☆	陈红风		上海中医药大学	
14	中医妇科学☆	冯晓玲	张婷婷	黑龙江中医药大学	上海中医药大学
15	中医儿科学☆	赵　霞	李新民	南京中医药大学	天津中医药大学
16	中医骨伤科学☆	黄桂成	王拥军	南京中医药大学	上海中医药大学
17	中医眼科学	彭清华		湖南中医药大学	
18	中医耳鼻咽喉科学	刘　蓬		广州中医药大学	
19	中医急诊学☆	刘清泉	方邦江	首都医科大学	上海中医药大学
20	中医各家学说☆	尚　力	戴　铭	上海中医药大学	广西中医药大学
21	针灸学☆	梁繁荣	王　华	成都中医药大学	湖北中医药大学
22	推拿学☆	房　敏	王金贵	上海中医药大学	天津中医药大学
23	中医养生学	马烈光	章德林	成都中医药大学	江西中医药大学
24	中医药膳学	谢梦洲	朱天民	湖南中医药大学	成都中医药大学
25	中医食疗学	施洪飞	方　泓	南京中医药大学	上海中医药大学
26	中医气功学	章文春	魏玉龙	江西中医药大学	北京中医药大学
27	细胞生物学	赵宗江	高碧珍	北京中医药大学	福建中医药大学

序号	书名	主编		主编所在单位	
28	人体解剖学	邵水金		上海中医药大学	
29	组织学与胚胎学	周忠光	汪涛	黑龙江中医药大学	天津中医药大学
30	生物化学	唐炳华		北京中医药大学	
31	生理学	赵铁建	朱大诚	广西中医药大学	江西中医药大学
32	病理学	刘春英	高维娟	辽宁中医药大学	河北中医学院
33	免疫学基础与病原生物学	袁嘉丽	刘永琦	云南中医药大学	甘肃中医药大学
34	预防医学	史周华		山东中医药大学	
35	药理学	张硕峰	方晓艳	北京中医药大学	河南中医药大学
36	诊断学	詹华奎		成都中医药大学	
37	医学影像学	侯键	许茂盛	成都中医药大学	浙江中医药大学
38	内科学	潘涛	戴爱国	南京中医药大学	湖南中医药大学
39	外科学	谢建兴		广州中医药大学	
40	中西医文献检索	林丹红	孙玲	福建中医药大学	湖北中医药大学
41	中医疫病学	张伯礼	吕文亮	天津中医药大学	湖北中医药大学
42	中医文化学	张其成	臧守虎	北京中医药大学	山东中医药大学

（二）针灸推拿学专业

序号	书名	主编		主编所在单位	
43	局部解剖学	姜国华	李义凯	黑龙江中医药大学	南方医科大学
44	经络腧穴学☆	沈雪勇	刘存志	上海中医药大学	北京中医药大学
45	刺法灸法学☆	王富春	岳增辉	长春中医药大学	湖南中医药大学
46	针灸治疗学☆	高树中	冀来喜	山东中医药大学	山西中医药大学
47	各家针灸学说	高希言	王威	河南中医药大学	辽宁中医药大学
48	针灸医籍选读	常小荣	张建斌	湖南中医药大学	南京中医药大学
49	实验针灸学	郭义		天津中医药大学	
50	推拿手法学☆	周运峰		河南中医药大学	
51	推拿功法学☆	吕立江		浙江中医药大学	
52	推拿治疗学☆	井夫杰	杨永刚	山东中医药大学	长春中医药大学
53	小儿推拿学	刘明军	邰先桃	长春中医药大学	云南中医药大学

（三）中西医临床医学专业

序号	书名	主编		主编所在单位	
54	中外医学史	王振国	徐建云	山东中医药大学	南京中医药大学
55	中西医结合内科学	陈志强	杨文明	河北中医学院	安徽中医药大学
56	中西医结合外科学	何清湖		湖南中医药大学	
57	中西医结合妇产科学	杜惠兰		河北中医学院	
58	中西医结合儿科学	王雪峰	郑健	辽宁中医药大学	福建中医药大学
59	中西医结合骨伤科学	詹红生	刘军	上海中医药大学	广州中医药大学
60	中西医结合眼科学	段俊国	毕宏生	成都中医药大学	山东中医药大学
61	中西医结合耳鼻咽喉科学	张勤修	陈文勇	成都中医药大学	广州中医药大学
62	中西医结合口腔科学	谭劲		湖南中医药大学	

（四）中药学类专业

序号	书　名	主　编		主编所在单位	
63	中医学基础	陈　晶	程海波	黑龙江中医药大学	南京中医药大学
64	高等数学	李秀昌	邵建华	长春中医药大学	上海中医药大学
65	中医药统计学	何　雁		江西中医药大学	
66	物理学	章新友	侯俊玲	江西中医药大学	北京中医药大学
67	无机化学	杨怀霞	吴培云	河南中医药大学	安徽中医药大学
68	有机化学	林　辉		广州中医药大学	
69	分析化学（上）（化学分析）	张　凌		江西中医药大学	
70	分析化学（下）（仪器分析）	王淑美		广东药科大学	
71	物理化学	刘　雄	王颖莉	甘肃中医药大学	山西中医药大学
72	临床中药学☆	周祯祥	唐德才	湖北中医药大学	南京中医药大学
73	方剂学	贾　波	许二平	成都中医药大学	河南中医药大学
74	中药药剂学☆	杨　明		江西中医药大学	
75	中药鉴定学☆	康廷国	闫永红	辽宁中医药大学	北京中医药大学
76	中药药理学☆	彭　成		成都中医药大学	
77	中药拉丁语	李　峰	马　琳	山东中医药大学	天津中医药大学
78	药用植物学☆	刘春生	谷　巍	北京中医药大学	南京中医药大学
79	中药炮制学☆	钟凌云		江西中医药大学	
80	中药分析学☆	梁生旺	张　彤	广东药科大学	上海中医药大学
81	中药化学☆	匡海学	冯卫生	黑龙江中医药大学	河南中医药大学
82	中药制药工程原理与设备	周长征		山东中医药大学	
83	药事管理学☆	刘红宁		江西中医药大学	
84	本草典籍选读	彭代银	陈仁寿	安徽中医药大学	南京中医药大学
85	中药制药分离工程	朱卫丰		江西中医药大学	
86	中药制药设备与车间设计	李　正		天津中医药大学	
87	药用植物栽培学	张永清		山东中医药大学	
88	中药资源学	马云桐		成都中医药大学	
89	中药产品与开发	孟宪生		辽宁中医药大学	
90	中药加工与炮制学	王秋红		广东药科大学	
91	人体形态学	武煜明	游言文	云南中医药大学	河南中医药大学
92	生理学基础	于远望		陕西中医药大学	
93	病理学基础	王　谦		北京中医药大学	

（五）护理学专业

序号	书　名	主　编		主编所在单位	
94	中医护理学基础	徐桂华	胡　慧	南京中医药大学	湖北中医药大学
95	护理学导论	穆　欣	马小琴	黑龙江中医药大学	浙江中医药大学
96	护理学基础	杨巧菊		河南中医药大学	
97	护理专业英语	刘红霞	刘　娅	北京中医药大学	湖北中医药大学
98	护理美学	余雨枫		成都中医药大学	
99	健康评估	阚丽君	张玉芳	黑龙江中医药大学	山东中医药大学

序号	书 名	主 编		主编所在单位	
100	护理心理学	郝玉芳		北京中医药大学	
101	护理伦理学	崔瑞兰		山东中医药大学	
102	内科护理学	陈 燕	孙志岭	湖南中医药大学	南京中医药大学
103	外科护理学	陆静波	蔡恩丽	上海中医药大学	云南中医药大学
104	妇产科护理学	冯 进	王丽芹	湖南中医药大学	黑龙江中医药大学
105	儿科护理学	肖洪玲	陈偶英	安徽中医药大学	湖南中医药大学
106	五官科护理学	喻京生		湖南中医药大学	
107	老年护理学	王 燕	高 静	天津中医药大学	成都中医药大学
108	急救护理学	吕 静	卢根娣	长春中医药大学	上海中医药大学
109	康复护理学	陈锦秀	汤继芹	福建中医药大学	山东中医药大学
110	社区护理学	沈翠珍	王诗源	浙江中医药大学	山东中医药大学
111	中医临床护理学	裘秀月	刘建军	浙江中医药大学	江西中医药大学
112	护理管理学	全小明	柏亚妹	广州中医药大学	南京中医药大学
113	医学营养学	聂 宏	李艳玲	黑龙江中医药大学	天津中医药大学

（六）公共课

序号	书 名	主 编		主编所在单位	
114	中医学概论	储全根	胡志希	安徽中医药大学	湖南中医药大学
115	传统体育	吴志坤	邵玉萍	上海中医药大学	湖北中医药大学
116	科研思路与方法	刘 涛	商洪才	南京中医药大学	北京中医药大学

（七）中医骨伤科学专业

序号	书 名	主 编		主编所在单位	
117	中医骨伤科学基础	李 楠	李 刚	福建中医药大学	山东中医药大学
118	骨伤解剖学	侯德才	姜国华	辽宁中医药大学	黑龙江中医药大学
119	骨伤影像学	栾金红	郭会利	黑龙江中医药大学	河南中医药大学洛阳平乐正骨学院
120	中医正骨学	冷向阳	马 勇	长春中医药大学	南京中医药大学
121	中医筋伤学	周红海	于 栋	广西中医药大学	北京中医药大学
122	中医骨病学	徐展望	郑福增	山东中医药大学	河南中医药大学
123	创伤急救学	毕荣修	李无阴	山东中医药大学	河南中医药大学洛阳平乐正骨学院
124	骨伤手术学	童培建	曾意荣	浙江中医药大学	广州中医药大学

（八）中医养生学专业

序号	书 名	主 编		主编所在单位	
125	中医养生文献学	蒋力生	王 平	江西中医药大学	湖北中医药大学
126	中医治未病学概论	陈涤平		南京中医药大学	